"Dr. Kradjian has put together an account which is *must* reading for anyone interested in the control of breast cancer. His long experience as a surgeon, combined with his careful analysis of scientific research on the dietary control of breast cancer, has produced a superb story worth reading. His challenge to science and medicine is profound and reliable."
— T. COLIN CAMPBELL, Ph.D., Jacob Gould
Schurman Professor of Biochemistry,
and Director, China Diet Health Project,
Cornell University

"2500 years ago, Hippocrates said: Let food be thy medicine. Dr. Kradjian—this is the beginning, you have paved the way for a prevention plan. It's time women hear all the options and realize the true value of food. And it's time we had a book like this! Bravo!"
— MATUSCHKA, artist, activist, macrobiotic practitioner,
and breast cancer Thriver

"As a breast cancer patient for whom prevention information was too late, I urge you to read this book. You owe it to yourself and to every woman you know to learn and share this information in order to stop the breast cancer epidemic."
— RUTH E. HEIDRICH, Ph.D., twelve year breast cancer
survivor, Ironman Triathlete and author of
*A Race for Life*

"The definitive guide to the beneficial use of diet in protecting women from breast cancer. Women who choose to follow Dr. Kradjian's program can make strides in protecting themsevles from this dread disease."
— SUSAN M. LARK, M.D., author of *The Menopause
Self-Help Book* and *The Estrogen Decision*

"We women have to wake up to the epidemic among us. The guidelines that Dr. Kradjian elucidates can reduce not only rates of breast cancer, but also rates of heart disease, stroke, osteoporosis, and many other cancers as well. As a gynecological cancer surgeon, it breaks my heart to see so many women developing diseases and cancers that are potentially preventable by improving our diet and exercise routines. Dr. Kradjian's guidelines are a diet for our lives!"
—KATHERINE A. O'HANLAN, M.D., Associate Director, Gynecological Cancer Section, Stanford University Medical Center

"Nutrition through a very low-fat diet is the only logical and safe approach to prevent breast cancer. A very low-fat diet can prevent other serious disorders such as coronary artery disease. Dr. Kradjian's book emphasizes this and tells us that we must do more than simply detect this lethal disease as early as possible, we must prevent it!"
—WILLIAM E. CONNOR, M.D., Professor of Medicine and Clinical Nutrition, Oregon Health Sciences University
—SONJA L. CONNOR, M.S., R.D., Research Associate, Professor of Clinical Nutrition, Oregon Health Sciences University

# SAVE YOURSELF from BREAST CANCER

Robert M. Kradjian, M.D.

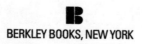

BERKLEY BOOKS, NEW YORK

This is an original edition from the Berkley Publishing Group and has never been previously published.

SAVE YOURSELF FROM BREAST CANCER

A Berkley Book / published by arrangement with the author

PRINTING HISTORY
Berkley trade paperback edition / November 1994

ISBN: 0-425-14390-2

BERKLEY®
Berkley Books are published by The Berkley Publishing Group, 200 Madison Avenue, New York, New York 10016. BERKLEY and the "B" design are trademarks belonging to Berkley Publishing Corporation.

PRINTED IN THE UNITED STATES OF AMERICA

10  9  8  7  6  5  4  3  2  1

This book is respectfully dedicated to my breast cancer patients. They have taught me much about love for life and personal courage.

"To ward off disease or recover health, men as a rule find it easier to depend on healers than to attempt the more difficult task of living wisely."
—RENE DUBOS,
Mirage of Health (1959)

"It often happens that the universal belief of one age, a belief from which no one was free or could be free without an extraordinary effort of genius or courage, becomes to a subsequent age, so palpable an absurdity that the only difference is, to imagine how such an idea could ever have appeared credible."
—JOHN STUART MILL

"One should not walk through the world wearing blinders."
—ALBERT EINSTEIN

# Acknowledgments

*T*his is to acknowledge the continuing support, encouragement, and contributions of my wife, Christine. Without her this book could not have been written.

My thanks to the following friends and colleagues who reviewed the manuscript and made valuable suggestions: Jeff Gee, M.D., an excellent primary-care physician; Monica Flores, who gave me the reaction of a young woman confronted with the problem of breast cancer prevention. Harry O'Neil provided an academic orientation and the data on the diet of the ancients. Carroll Bellis, M.D., surgical pioneer and scholar, and William Yannuzzi, music director of the Baltimore Opera, read the manuscript from the literary point of view. William Harris, M.D., a thorough student of the interactions between nutrition and health, was the first to scientifically explain to me the benefits of proper nutrition while we were volunteer civilian physicians in Vietnam nearly thirty years ago. Leonard Shlain, M.D., offered early encouragement for the book. Special thanks to my excellent agent, Robert Stricker; to Kate Ross and Georgia Hughes, who provided not only editorial help, but a woman's perspective; to Olga Veit, a wonderful patient and an expert in language; to Janice Perlman-Stites for assistance with the chapter notes; and to my editor, Elizabeth Beier, who shaped the book and who had unswerving faith in the project.

# Contents

# CHARTS FOR *SAVE YOURSELF FROM BREAST CANCER*

# Author's Note

Medical and scientific research has shown that there are strong links between nutrition and breast cancer. The information in this book summarizes some of that data. It is my conclusion that diet is the primary factor in the genesis of breast cancer, while heredity accounts for only a small percentage of cases. Environmental pollutants are possibly cofactors. The role of stress and electromagnetic fields is not thought to be critical.

This book is not intended to serve as a source of information regarding the treatment of breast cancer. Diet alone is not recommended for this condition, although I believe that it is a powerful adjunct to conventional treatment. Any woman with this serious disorder should seek medical consultation and place herself under the care of physicians. Breast lumps, other breast abnormalities, or abnormal mammograms should be promptly investigated and appropriate therapy initiated. Persons changing their diet while on medication may need to alter dosages with the guidance of their physicians.

This book does not describe a "get well quick" scheme.

It is a book about prevention and prevention requires time. My prevention plan is relatively easy to implement with proper motivation. A great number of women are successful in following this plan, and in so doing enjoy a degree of protection from breast cancer as well as a number of other serious diseases. They also report an increased feeling of well-being as well as enhanced energy levels.

A book can be a seed, and a seed can provide growth. It is my wish that the most precious growth of all, human life, will be prolonged by the simple message contained here.

### Sources

I have used four main sources for the information presented in this book. The first—and by far the most important—was the world's scientific literature, chiefly current, but also from the past eight decades. I have used standard medical and surgical journals and books, as well as scientific publications from other disciplines. The National Library of Medicine Database was particularly useful. In all, more than seven thousand articles were reviewed. A second source was information available to any American: magazines, newspapers, television, and radio. A third source was governmental publications, and fourth, personal communication with medical experts, my patients, industry workers, and government officials. Finally, I relied on my own medical and surgical experience over the past thirty years.

—Robert M. Kradjian, M.D., Breast Surgeon
Spring 1994

# Foreword

*Save Yourself from Breast Cancer* is an opportunity for women to take control of their health. Dr. Robert Kradjian edited mountains of data into a readable reference text for women who want to be proactive in their health destiny.

The author is one of a thoughtful group of health professionals who increasingly question the dogma that breast cancer is in the genes.

He carefully outlines the present establishment position of only emphasizing early diagnosis. This is an impossible dilemma for women. Breast cancer in its earliest form has been present eight to ten years with an opportunity to metastasize long before it can be detected. The answer to this challenge is to teach women how they can avoid breast cancer in the first place. This is the only answer to the epidemic of breast cancer which continues out of control. No matter how many times an early diagnosis is made, it does nothing to eliminate new breast cancers in the coming generations. That will only come about through the comprehensive lifestyle changes which Dr. Kradjian defines.

Why should he write this book? Why rock the boat? Why risk being ridiculed by the establishment? It is worth it because of the enormous satisfaction and pride of accomplishment in trying to educate women so they may avoid this disfiguring and all-too-often fatal disease. A number of us as surgeons have realized the futility of dealing, by strictly mechanical means, with disease which is of molecular and biochemical origin. Dr. Kradjian's powers of observation of this disease during a lifetime of experience and his awareness of the literature on breast cancer have been the crucible of knowledge that is apparent in every chapter.

The sequence of his chapters brings order, compelling logic, and common sense to his position that it is the western diet—with its emphasis on animal protein, fat, lack of fiber, and lack of vegetarian products—which accounts for the epidemic of breast cancer.

Dr. Kradjian carefully outlines the arguments for his position. The cultural difference in breast cancer incidence with migration patterns is well documented. He clearly defines the risk of obesity, increased bodily estrogen, lack of exercise, and the immune suppressive tendency of a high-fat diet. The reader can easily appreciate the lucid confirmation of that fat hypothesis as revealed in the animal studies which are reviewed.

It is an honor to write this foreword for *Save Yourself from Breast Cancer*. This book reflects the knowledge of a "hands on" physician who has the wisdom, caring, and energy to show women how they may best protect themselves from developing breast cancer.

—Caldwell B. Esselstyn, Jr., M.D.
Head, Section of Thyroid and Parathyroid Surgery;
Staff Surgeon, Department of General Surgery;
Former Chairman, Breast Cancer Task Force;
Director, 1st National Conference on the
Elimination of Coronary Artery Disease;
The Cleveland Clinic Foundation,
Cleveland, Ohio

# Breast Cancer:
# The Neglected Epidemic

*B*reast cancer is common, dangerous, and on the increase. It is the most feared cancer in America.

The breast is a powerful external symbol of femininity, motherhood, and beauty. When a woman is diagnosed with breast cancer, the emotional shock is much greater than with more neutral areas of the body.

Our leading health agencies and medical authorities have told women that their best defense against breast cancer is an excellent program of early detection. I believe in this approach and teach a comprehensive detection program both in my medical practice and in my lectures. However, early detection is often not enough. Over thirty years of surgical practice, I have treated many women who faithfully followed all of the recommended advice, yet were found to have tumors that were beyond medical control at the time of earliest possible detection. We urgently need a program of prevention as well as early detection. It is far better to prevent a disease than to attempt to cure it. Early detection attempts, without prevention, have not succeeded. *The overall mortality rates for breast cancer have not improved from 1930 to the pres-*

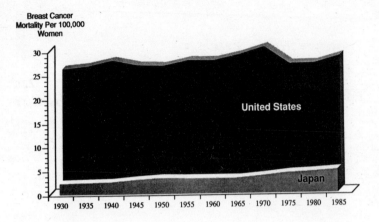

**Breast Cancer Mortality**
**U.S. vs. Japan**

1. Wynder E L. et al. Comparative Epidemiology of Cancer Between the United States and Japan. Cancer February 1, 1991, pgs 746-763.
2. *Clincal Oncology*, American Cancer Society 1991, pg 6.

*ent*. In fact, there is a very gradual worsening trend. Breast cancer has become a neglected epidemic.

Despite the fact that the medical establishment claims to support prevention, it has repeatedly described dietary efforts as faulty and has rejected preventive programs well within our reach. I believe that this attitude is costing lives every day. In *Save Yourself from Breast Cancer*, I've sidestepped the official view and described a practical prevention program for women who need it now.

Breast cancer has always been a serious concern, but in the last twenty years the number of reported cases has soared. In the United States at the turn of the century, breast cancer was a relatively rare disease. Now it is the most common cancer among American women and the second most frequent cause of death from cancer (behind only lung cancer).

Why has breast cancer become more common and why is it increasingly affecting younger women?

## Interpreting the Statistics

The 1994 breast cancer projections tell us that 182,000 U.S. women will be diagnosed with the disease during that year. Of those women, 46,000 will die.[1] One statistic rarely explored is the estimated 1.5 million family members who have survived the loss of a loved one to breast cancer. Breast cancer involves very young women, in sharp contradistinction to all the other common cancers. It is the leading cause of all mortality in women 40–49 years of age. And 24 percent of all breast cancer deaths occur in women who are 50 years of age or younger at the time of diagnosis. This is what leaves many more young children, husbands, and other relatives to grieve. A breast cancer death takes an average of twenty years from a woman's life. This means nearly a *million* years of women's lives are lost to breast cancer each year in the United States.

Breast cancer is the cancer for which the most X-ray examinations are made. It is the cancer for which the most biopsies are performed. It is the cancer for which the most radiation therapy is given. No other cancer is treated with so much chemotherapy. No other cancer requires as much hormonal therapy. No other cancer—with the exception of skin cancer—is so often discovered by the patient herself. Despite years of study, there is still no unanimity regarding treatment. We do not even know with certainty the prognosis or the survival prospects for newly diagnosed cases.

In 1991 we were told that one woman in nine would eventually develop breast cancer in this country. This figure was based on a cumulative risk until age eighty-five.[2] Au-

## Odds of Developing Breast Cancer by Age
### (American Women)

| Age | Odds of Developing Breast Cancer One In: |
|---|---|
| 25 | 19,608 |
| 30 | 2,525 |
| 35 | 622 |
| 40 | 217 |
| 45 | 93 |
| **50** | **50** |
| 55 | 33 |
| 60 | 24 |
| 65 | 17 |
| 70 | 14 |
| 75 | 11 |
| 80 | 10 |
| 85 | 9 |
| 95+ | 8 |

SEER Program of National Cancer Society, the National Cancer Institute, and the American Cancer Society. From NABCO, 1993.

thorities now say *one in eight*, during a woman's entire lifetime, is the correct figure.

More than 12 percent of all women in America will eventually develop breast cancer according to this method of measurement. The risk of developing cancer for each consecutive ten-year period is computed until a woman reaches the theoretical age of 110 years. Each of these ten-year segments has its own risk, and the risk for each segment is added, or becomes cumulative. For a thirty-five-year-old woman the risk is low—approximately 1 in 622—but by age forty, it is 1 in 217. At fifty, it is 1 in 50, and by age sixty, it is only about 1 in 24. It is not until a woman reaches the age of seventy that her risk is more than 7 percent, or 1 in 14. At eighty, it is 1 in 10. The lifetime, cumulative risk therefore approaches one in eight, or approximately 12 percent of women only toward the end of a long life (ninety-five or more years).

Although cancer statistics usually contain adjustments for the number of women living to older ages, there is no doubt that increased longevity has subjected many additional thousands of older women to the risk of breast cancer.

Our current projections indicate that of the women developing breast cancer, at least 25 percent will eventually die of the disease, even with the most optimistic projections.[3]

However, some others describe the situation as much worse. In the Netherlands, J. G. Klijn and his associates[4] tell us that at least half of their patients with breast cancer will ultimately die of that disease. One respected researcher, Dr. C. Barber Mueller, professor emeritus of surgery from McMaster University at Hamilton, Ontario, Canada, feels that the true number is even greater than that described by the Dutch investigators.[5] He followed 3,558 breast cancer patients from upstate New York for nineteen years. At the end of that time, 1,660 of those women were dead and 88 percent of them had died of breast cancer! Dr. Mueller believes that if all breast cancer patients are followed carefully until the end of their lives, breast cancer is by far their major cause of death. He feels that modern statisticians, researchers, and clinicians attempt artificially to improve their results by selecting favorable, early cases and unrealistically short follow-up periods. Less favorable cases with advanced disease and women with late recurrence of tumor are thus excluded from these reports. This method is called *fixed-time survivorship*, and is usually expressed in five- and ten-year survival rates. Such projections give better results than the *life-table analysis* method Dr. Mueller recommends. This method requires determination of the annual status of all patients and uses all data available, even including data on patients who may be lost to follow-up.

Dr. Mueller is not alone in this gloomy assessment. Drs. David Plotkin and Francis Blankenberg describe a similar statistical picture.[6] They write that five-year survival without evidence of recurrence is a widely quoted, but inaccurate, definition of cure. They note that the survival of a patient is measured from the time of the initial tissue or pathologic diagnosis. Any technique that leads to earlier sampling of tissue and confirmation of the diagnosis will provide an improved specific term survival without necessarily altering the curability of the breast cancer. Using a more sensitive and accurate method of evaluating mortality called the *relative survival method*, an excess of mortality due to breast cancer has been observed up to forty years from the time of diagnosis. In addition to the studies of C. B. Mueller mentioned above, large-scale registry-based studies in Norway[7] and England lead to the dismal conclusion that if a group of women diagnosed with breast cancer are followed up until the end of their lives, the odds are that approximately 80 percent of them will die of breast cancer![8] The remaining 20 percent, of course, die of "old age" or non–breast cancer causes. The Mueller study also clearly shows that the death rate from breast cancer is far higher in the youngest women. His conclusion is that the older women died of a competing disease, and had they lived long enough, they would possibly also have been claimed by breast cancer.

A study in England followed a small group of 704 breast cancer patients for nearly thirty-one years. The numbers of deaths from cancer of the breast after twenty-five years was fifteen times the number that would be expected in a normal population.[9]

Additional long-term studies from Scandinavia and Europe tell the same story. In Sweden, 14,731 women with breast cancer were followed for five to eighteen years. An excess of mortality from breast cancer persisted throughout the entire study when the breast cancer patients were compared with the normal, matched women in the population.

Deaths from breast cancer can occur up to thirty years from the time of original treatment, and in rare cases even longer. The longest interval between treatment and recurrence of breast cancer that I found in the scientific literature was in a French report. A ninety-nine-year-old patient had a recurrence of tumor fifty years after mastectomy. Because of the very long natural history of breast cancer, most researchers content themselves with short-term markers, such as the five-year cure rate, and the *disease-free interval*. This can provide a falsely optimistic picture.

Breast cancer is a long-acting disease, but what about its incidence? Is breast cancer truly increasing? Unfortunately, it seems to be. Let's go back in American history to 1840. The estimated breast cancer rate then was 15 to 20 per 100,000 women. By 1880 this had risen to 50, and by 1900 to 64 per 100,000. There was a slow and steady rise until midcentury, when the rate of increase turned sharply upward. There was another surge in breast cancer diagnosis in 1974, and by 1980 the rate was 84.8 per 100,000, rising to the low nineties by 1985. The rate of increase remained quite substantial at 4 to 6 percent per year. By 1987, the rate had further increased to 112.4.[10] Currently the annual increase is estimated at 2 to 3 percent[11] and the rate per 100,000 is around 120.[12] All this happened during an era in which the president of the United States had "declared war on cancer" and billions of dollars had been spent on research.

Trends in breast cancer mortality in Connecticut were studied at Yale University in 1991.[13] The study confirmed a continuing increase in breast cancer over a ninety-year period.

The Kaiser Foundation physicians in the Portland, Oregon, area have been following their health plan patients

**Breast Cancer Incidence, U.S. Women**

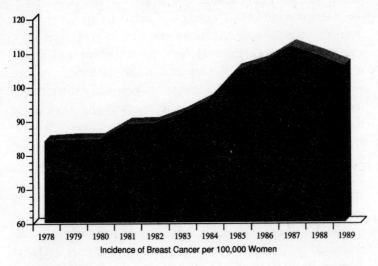

Incidence of Breast Cancer per 100,000 Women

1. National Cancer Institute 1990.
2. CA January/February 1993, Vol. 43, No. 1, pg. 30

for many years. They noted a 45 percent increase in breast cancer from 1960 to 1985. Since they already had a comprehensive health surveillance program in place, they concluded that only a small amount of that increase was due to improved or more frequent mammographic studies.[14]

I recall being distressed at learning in medical school during the late 1950s that breast cancer would eventually involve one out of every twenty American women. When I wrote a patient-information booklet on breast cancer in 1978, I was even more disturbed to learn that the incidence had increased to one in fourteen American women. Every time I updated the booklet for subsequent editions the situation had worsened. From one in twelve in 1982, it increased to one in ten by 1989. And now, in 1994, it is estimated that one of every eight American women will develop breast cancer should she live to be one hundred years of age.

## How We Got Here

How did breast cancer take such a firm hold in the United States? What are the barriers that have prevented us from changing the course of these grim statistics?

To begin with, the search for the causes of breast cancer is and always has been minimal. Most research has centered on molecular biology, genetics, and on treatment or diagnostic techniques. But it is becoming increasingly clear to many observers that breast cancer is in many ways an environmental disease, and may therefore be preventable.[15] Yet the American medical establishment has only partially informed the women of America about any possibility of breast cancer prevention. The result is that women who wish to protect themselves do not have the information at their disposal to do so.

Additionally, much of what women do know about this disease is based on "myth" and misinformation, which must be dispelled before a clear understanding of breast cancer prevention can emerge. Myths often contain elements of truth, but there is much more to be considered. Let's take a look at some of the more common myths regarding breast cancer and evaluate each.

## Breast Cancer Myths

• **Myth 1: Breast cancer cannot be prevented since its cause is not known.**
Truth: All diseases have causes, and common diseases have

common causes. Breast cancer causes include genetic susceptibility, a high-fat/low-fiber diet, alcohol use, obesity, and a sedentary lifestyle.

• **Myth 2: Breast cancer randomly strikes women; all American women are at risk.**
Truth: Two basic forces push women toward breast cancer: heredity and the environment. Heredity cannot be changed, but women can change environmental factors.

• **Myth 3: A woman's best "defense" is to detect the breast cancer early.**
Truth: Early detection is obviously desirable, but breast cancer is not being controlled by early detection alone. The best defense is prevention.

• **Myth 4: Nearly all who find breast cancer "early" will be cured.**
Truth: Early detection is best. Too few American women avail themselves of detection procedures. Unfortunately, in many cases breast cancer has already spread when first detected.

• **Myth 5: Breast cancer is rapidly increasing, and no one knows why.**
Truth: Some of the increase is due to improved mammographic detection, but environmental factors are clearly to blame. Among these, a high-fat/low-fiber diet is the chief suspect.

• **Myth 6: Postmenopausal hormone therapy cannot contribute to breast cancer.**
Truth: Depending on the dose, type, and duration of hormone therapy, there is an increased risk of breast and uterine cancer.

• **Myth 7: Without postmenopausal estrogen, I will certainly develop osteoporosis or heart disease.**

Truth: There are other ways, chiefly dietary modification, to combat osteoporosis and heart disease. Estrogen therapy is best reserved for troublesome symptoms and short-term use.

• **Myth 8: Research will produce a breakthrough and cure breast cancer.**

Truth: Diseases are eliminated by prevention, immunization, public health policies, and civil engineering. Diseases are not eliminated by treatment alone, and rarely by high-tech research.

• **Myth 9: The government will protect me.**

Truth: The government has not developed an effective policy to combat breast cancer.

• **Myth 10: Modern surgery, radiation, and chemotherapy are highly effective and advanced tools in the battle against breast cancer.**

Truth: Breast cancer therapies are harsh and relatively ineffective. The death rates have remained unchanged for fifty years.

• **Myth 11: Breast cancer patients fit a specific psychological profile. Stress causes breast cancer.**

Truth: All psychological types can develop breast cancer. The rich American diet is at fault, not American women. There is no convincing evidence that stress causes breast cancer.

• **Myth 12: Caffeine causes breast cancer.**

Truth: There is no evidence that caffeine causes breast cancer, and very little evidence that it contributes significantly to "fibrocystic disease."

• **Myth 13: Trauma (injury) causes breast cancer.**

Truth: There is no evidence that this is true.

• **Myth 14: Electromagnetic fields cause breast cancer.**

Truth: At present, there is no convincing evidence that electromagnetic fields are a serious hazard.

• **Myth 15: If a breast lump is painful, it can't be cancer.**

Truth: While most breast cancers are painless, tenderness is present in a minority of cases.

The medical establishment's current approach is based on early detection, treatment, and research. It is a proper approach, but an incomplete one. Early detection is often not early enough. Even when women follow all the recommended procedures, if breast cancer develops, it too often is detected in an advanced stage. Mammography is our best early-detection device, yet only a relatively few women avail themselves of it. A 1991 survey in San Diego determined that only 15 to 20 percent of women fifty years of age and older had ever had a mammogram.[16] Not only is mammography not as efficient as we would like, this study tells us that it is also underutilized.

It is important to remember that not all breast cancers show up on mammograms. Even the most enthusiastic supporter of mammography will admit that a 5-to-10-percent "false negative" rate exists. These are instances where breast cancer is present within the breast, but even a properly made and interpreted mammographic film does not reveal it. This by definition is a false-negative result. Some tumors are simply too soft, have the same consistency as the remainder of the breast tissue, contain no calcium (which shows up readily on an X ray), are too small, or in some other way do not appear on the film.

Surgery, chemotherapy, and radiation therapy are current weapons in the battle against breast cancer, but these are crude, harsh tools. They have side effects that are unacceptable to many and often are ineffective. Cure rates for breast cancer have remained static over many decades. Yet most medical professionals maintain a deep belief in these therapies. Research, although providing fascinating insights into biological processes, has given working doctors very little in the way of new, truly effective tools against breast cancer. We need a new approach in defending ourselves from this disease. We need prevention.

# 2

## How Breast Cancer Begins: Current Beliefs

*T*here is a great deal we do not know about breast cancer. However, what we do know about the beginnings of breast cancer provides a basis for understanding the breast cancer riddle.

Cancer is an uncontrolled growth of abnormal cells that has the dangerous capability to spread to distant parts of one's body by way of the bloodstream or another circulation system, the lymphatic system. It is now believed that at least two distinct stages are involved in cancer growth. The first is *initiation* and the second is *promotion*.

We have little idea how human breast cancers start or are initiated. But we do know that the basis of cancer is as follows: *Every minute ten million cells divide in the human body.*[17] They almost always divide in the correct manner, governed by incredibly complex controls. However, on the exceedingly rare occasions when the controls fail, initiation may occur, and cancer may develop. We know that initiators can be cancer-causing agents that damage a cell's genetic material, triggering the first growth of cancer. The initiation event may take place many years before the development of cancer, and it often represents a multistep process. For example, radiation to the necks of children can initiate the development of thyroid cancer decades later. In another example, the fertility hormone DES, given in the 1950s to young women who later became mothers, initiated the development of genital cancers in their adolescent daughters and even testicular cancers in their sons. Chemicals, infectious agents, even heredity can cause initiation.

Initiators can also act as promoters. Promoters are substances that are necessary for the growth of tumors. Initiation tends to be a quickly induced and permanent process. Promotion is a slow process that may stretch out over many years. Promotion causes cancer cells to multiply once they have been initiated. Dietary fat can act both as an initiator and as a promoter by acting directly on the cell membranes and the cell's genetic material, the DNA. Dietary fat can also contribute to cancer by altering the hormonal environment of the body's cells. Unlike initiation, promotion can be switched on or off by a large number of forces. Examples of such forces would be diet, vitamins, hormones, other medications, chemicals, alcohol, and the status of the immune system.

Any hope we have for reducing the probabilities of developing cancer lies in identifying and eliminating the initiating and promoting factors while, at the same time, increasing a friendly group of factors called *antipromoters*. Antipromoters can retard the growth of tumors. They include dietary fiber; vitamins A, C, E, and three specific groups of food: *cruciferous vegetables* (broccoli, cabbage, Brussels sprouts, radishes, turnips, collard greens, and cauliflower); the *protease inhibitors* (soybeans, garbanzos, lima, and other beans); and the foods high in *beta carotenes* (carrots, sweet potatoes, yams, yellow and green vegetables, and yellow or orange fruits). The possible role of vitamins, especially retinoic acid, a substance related to vitamin A, seems promising and is being investigated intensively. A National Cancer Institute–Chinese study on vitamin supplementation was announced on September 14, 1993, and published in the *Journal of the National Cancer Institute*. Researchers found that 29,584 persons randomly selected to take vitamin E and selenium on a daily basis for five years had an overall reduction in cancer of 13 percent. The considerable importance of dietary fiber in reducing breast cancer potential is also recognized by nearly all investigators.

For many, doctors and nondoctors alike, it is unsettling to realize that medical therapies are not all-powerful, and that simple efforts we make at home can be of great value in preventing disease. But using what we currently know about dietary promoters and antipromoters could make the crucial difference between developing or not developing breast cancer.

## What About Genetics?

Genetic factors are of great importance in the development of breast cancer. Some investigators feel that almost every disease is either caused by, or strongly influenced by, genetics. Who can argue against this? Among working physicians, this is a common belief. "It's all in a woman's genes," is often heard when physicians discuss breast cancer. But is it true?

Genes are the basic units of heredity located on the twenty-three pairs of chromosomes found in all human cells. Each individual cell contains 50,000 to 100,000 of these genes. The genes are composed of an acid found in the nucleus (center) of a cell; hence, the term *nucleic acid*, or *deoxyribonucleic acid (DNA)*. DNA is the genetic material of all higher organisms in nature. Think of the chromosomes and genes as tiny computer chips that program and control the reproduction and the vital functions of each cell. They also determine the thousands of traits that result in each individual's uniqueness.

We know that there is a small subset of women, probably one half of one percent of all breast cancer patients, who have inherited a specific gene that confers a very high risk for the development of breast cancer. It has been tentatively named the BRCA 1 (breast cancer) gene. This has been localized on chromosome 17q21, and attempts at "mapping" the gene and cloning it are in progress. Although this sounds ominous, it is important to keep a proper perspective on the magnitude of this particular inherited susceptibility problem. Only one in two hundred women to one in four hundred (approximately 600,000 women in the United States) have this genetic susceptibility to breast cancer.[18] This gives any individual woman a one half of one percent (0.5%) chance, or less, of having this trait. Even if you do have the trait, it is not absolutely inevitable that you will develop breast cancer. At age forty, your chances of developing breast cancer would be 16 percent; by age fifty, it would be much greater—58 percent. Even at eighty years of age, 15 percent of women with this rare and highly dangerous genetic trait will not develop breast cancer.

The effect of diet on this small group of women is unknown. Will a low-fat diet reduce the number who will develop breast cancer? It may, but I seriously doubt that it will totally eliminate the possibility. (An intriguing but unproved possibility is that the "irreducible minimum" of breast cancer that we seem to find in the very low-incidence areas of the world may chiefly represent women with the BRCA 1 gene. If that proposition proved to be the case, it would establish that very low-fat diets prevented breast cancer in all except those with the BRCA 1 gene!) For the overwhelming majority of the remaining women, the 199 out of 200, the maximum lifetime risk of an American woman for developing breast cancer is about 12 percent. Thus, the evidence indicates that breast cancer is *not* primarily a genetic disease, though, as we shall see, it *is* a *familial* disease. It has been estimated that less than 3 to 5 percent of breast cancer is strictly hereditary.

It may surprise you to learn that in every survey of breast cancer patients, *about 80 percent of them will have no blood relatives with breast cancer*! Doctors call this a *negative family history for breast cancer*. This consistent finding, along with the substantial and steady increases in incidence, *makes a purely genetic causation for breast cancer highly unlikely.* Genetic changes also tend to be glacially slow. It is a very odd genetic disorder when one's ancestors have the disease less than 20 percent of the time.

One of the best ways to study the effects of genetics on breast cancer is through observations of *identical twins.* There are some 2.5 million twins in the United States with 33,000 more arriving each year—about one of every 250 births. Identical, or monozygotic, twins are approximately a third of the twin total. Identical twins are as close to each other, genetically, as any two human beings can be. Yet when groups of female twins (where one has developed breast cancer) are studied, a surprising fact emerges. Fewer than 6 percent of the remaining twins will develop breast cancer! If breast cancer is primarily a genetic disease, as many believe, why wouldn't all—or at least most—of the remaining twins develop breast cancer? This is called *lack of concordance* by geneticists and is a very powerful clue to the essentially non-genetic nature of breast cancer. That is to say, the disease is not transmitted in the DNA and the RNA of the germ plasm at the time of conception. It is also of interest that recent twin studies tell us that what was previously considered to be a genetic origin of many diseases has been exaggerated.[19]

An important study with practical implications came from Denmark and assessed the relative contribution of genetics as compared to environment in adopted children born from 1924 to 1926.[20] Genetics was found to be more important than environment in vascular disease (mainly coronary disease and strokes). If either biological parent died from vascular disease before age fifty, the adoptees' risk of death from these causes was 4.5 times greater than average. But the *opposite* was true of cancer deaths. If an *adoptive* parent died of cancer, the risk of cancer in the adopted child was 5.16 times greater than average. If the biological parent died of cancer, there was only a 1.19 times greater chance of the adoptee dying of cancer! This clearly shows the tremendous impact of environment (in this case the family environment) on the subsequent development of cancer. Thus, genetics is less important than how the parents teach the child how to live. This helps to explain why breast cancer can be *familial* even when it is not *genetic*.

A large study of women was reported in the July 21, 1993, *Journal of the American Medical Association*[21] in which 117,988 women were followed for twelve years. Nearly 6 percent of the women reported that their mother had been diagnosed with breast cancer and just over one percent reported that their sister had been diagnosed with breast cancer. The overall increase of breast cancer in the group where the mother had breast cancer was just less than twice the average risk, and the risk for the group with an involved sister was over two times average risk. There was a 7 percent risk of breast cancer by age seventy if there was no family history of breast cancer at all. The conclusion was that within their study group, only 2.5 percent of breast cancer cases were attributable to family history. The women in the study were nurses, and had a higher rate of mammography surveillance than otherwise matched American women. Further, the women with a positive family history for breast cancer had an 8 percent higher mammography rate than the rest of the women, reflecting their heightened concern.

There is at least some good news concerning genetics

and breast cancer. Family history, one of the known risk factors, apparently renders some women *susceptible* to breast cancer, but the genes do not actually *cause* the disease as they do, for example, in Huntington's disease or cystic fibrosis. (A possible exception is the BRCA 1 gene discussed earlier.) This inherited susceptibility will have a minimal impact on an individual woman's health unless she is exposed to initiators and promoters: in brief, a high-fat/low-fiber diet. The genetic component and the environmental component are both needed to cause breast cancer. We now understand that breast cancer is the product of both our inheritance (unchangeable) and our environment (potentially changeable). Among all the environmental factors, diet is by far the most important.

I am certain that once you examine the evidence and begin to sort out fact from fiction, you will agree that breast cancer *can* be prevented.

# 3

## *Prevention Is the Answer*

*C*an something as simple as dietary change be a serious aid in combating a disease as deadly as breast cancer? I believe that it can.

Evidence informs us that women in many parts of the world are remarkably safe and seemingly protected from breast cancer. I see no logical or scientifically defensible reason why the factors that protect women in other parts of the world cannot be brought to American women. We import nearly everything else, why shouldn't we import a proven approach to breast cancer prevention? Why can't we analyze the protective features of other environments and adopt them for ourselves?

Some experts claim that the breast cancer seen, for example, in Asian women is "different" from that of American women and that Asian women are also genetically different. They can offer no scientific basis for this claim. These experts also are unable to explain the rapid increase in breast cancer cases observed among Asian women who come to America and adopt our style of living. In fact, most of the women on this planet live in a manner that is not only effective in reducing breast cancer risk, but also greatly reduces the probability of other "killer" diseases, including heart attacks, other cancers, strokes, and diabetes. For the men in their lives, prostate cancer—which is remarkably similar to breast cancer in both causes and incidence—responds to the *same* preventive measures.

I have been on the front lines of the surgical fight against this disease. I am not an armchair philosopher; I know breast cancer at first hand. Early in my career, I devoted four years to medicine with volunteer organizations, much of the time as chief of surgery on America's first peacetime hospital ship, the *S.S. Hope*. I learned something that most American surgeons never experience at first hand—namely, that cancer incidence varies tremendously among different countries in the world. Further, these differences seemed to be related to everyday choices—chiefly dietary choices—made by the people involved.

Here's an example from my own experience. In 1968 the *S.S. Hope* sailed to Colombo, Ceylon (now Sri Lanka), where we spent a year teaching medical students and residents and helping with the treatment of patients. I was privileged to be the chief of surgery for the project, and in my efforts to share the latest in American surgical techniques with the young doctors from their medical school, I asked them to select a suitable breast cancer patient to be brought to the hospital ship. When the doctors failed to present such a patient after several weeks, my request was met with: "But Dr. Kradjian, we haven't *had* a breast cancer patient." I reminded them that they had over five thousand outpatient visits a day to the huge Colombo General Hospital Outpatient Department and that they should have had several *dozen* breast cancer patients. They looked at me and silently shook their heads.

In 1968, I did not comprehend that *country of birth* was a strong risk factor for breast cancer—that a woman born in America was destined to a high breast cancer risk while a

Ceylonese-born woman was somehow protected. I believed *exactly* what I had been taught. My professors never told me that nutrition was important in the causation of disease except in rare and exotic deficiency diseases such as scurvy, pellagra, or beriberi. They were only beginning to open their minds to the possibility that saturated fat and cholesterol were of some importance in the development of heart disease. These were the early days of nutritional understanding.

After many weeks we finally got our breast cancer patient, the operation was performed, and the requisite lectures and teaching followed. We now know that breast cancer was, and still is, a rare disease in Sri Lanka compared with the United States and other Western countries. When a great pioneer in breast surgery, George Crile, Jr., came to Ceylon to visit our project, he also noticed that there were only a handful of breast cancer patients in the huge Colombo General Hospital. He assumed, as I had, that this was due only to a momentary lull in the usual stream of patients that an American or European surgeon would see in his or her clinic. For a fascinating account of the entire year that the *S.S. Hope* spent in Ceylon, see Dr. William B. Walsh's *Hope in the East*. [22](Included are photographs of me with my new bride, Christine, a talented cardiac-care nurse, who pioneered the setting up of Ceylon's first coronary intensive-care unit.)

Evidence such as this should at the very least open the discussion of the effect of diet on the development of breast cancer. The medical establishment, however, believes that a number of factors may be involved in the development of breast cancer and that these factors may operate in a complex series of stages. Breast cancer is thus said to be a *multifactorial disease*.

Every breast cancer expert has detailed knowledge of a long list of *risk factors* that is often recited in response to the question "What causes breast cancer?" The listing of risk factors is not the same as identifying a cause for breast cancer. This risk-factor approach has been passed on by the medical profession for many decades. By simply compiling and providing a list of factors, medical experts have avoided the more serious and difficult task of identifying the causes of this disease.

Despite this, the risk factors provided for breast cancer are important. A partial listing of these proven factors usually includes the following:

- A personal history of previous breast cancer
- A personal history of cancer of the ovary or uterus
- A family history, particularly with mother or sisters, less importantly with grandmothers, least with aunts and cousins (the effect is greater if the disease occurred before the menopause of the affected relative or was present in both breasts).
- Early menarche (onset of menstrual periods before age 12)
- Late menopause (after age 55)
- Age (more than 85 percent of breast cancers occur after the age of forty-five)
- Having no children, or having the first child after age thirty
- Not nursing one's children for four months or longer
- Benign breast disease, especially if that benign disease is atypical (tending toward malignancy) on biopsy
- Obesity
- Alcohol use
- Prolonged oral contraceptive usage
- Prolonged hormone replacement therapy
- Height (tallness)
- High-fat/low-fiber diet
- Exposure to strong radiation
- Affluence
- Urban living
- High educational status
- Being Caucasian

This is an impressive list, and even a useful one, but it does not establish the cause of breast cancer. Worse, a full 60 percent of breast cancer patients, and perhaps even as many as 70 percent, have none of these factors *except for the usual diet eaten by nearly all American women.* This is a crucial observation. When a disease seems to sweep across a country, there must be a nearly universal risk factor, and in the case of breast cancer, that seems to be chronically elevated estrogen levels. A rich diet emerges from this listing of risk factors as the key suspect in the causation of those elevated estrogen levels—and therefore breast cancer—among American women.

With the exception of diet, none of the above-listed risk factors can reasonably be expected to account for the huge variations in breast cancer incidence observed around the world.

As a practical matter, altering most of the other listed risk factors is simply beyond our control. For example, we can do nothing to change our family history. There are other factors that are potentially controllable, but not without a major dislocation or disruption in one's personal life. Only dietary change and reduction of obesity emerge as factors that can be changed by any woman, at any time, without harmful health consequences or personal upheaval.

Each time we eat a foodstuff, within minutes, molecules from that food enter or surround each of the *trillions* of cells in our body. By age sixty-five many humans have ingested *over 100,000 pounds* of food, making food our most profound, intimate, and decisive involvement with our environment.

All diseases have causes, yet sometimes we are unable fully to determine them. If we cannot learn the cause or causes of a disease, we should then make all reasonable attempts to learn as much as possible about the most likely causes, with special emphasis on those that are open to safe and appropriate change. Breast cancer is a common disease, and *common diseases have common causes*. The rich American diet, with its high dietary fat and low fiber level, is the primary common factor that is most likely to be the cause of the breast cancer explosion in the United States.

I can see no value in waiting until the entire breast cancer picture is fully clarified before taking action. Medical scientists have not done that in the past. The story of the conquest of cholera is an early example. Dr. John Snow, a London physician in the early 1800s, not only recognized but acted on the belief that cholera was transmitted by the drinking water from a single well. He directed that the handle be removed from the well's pump. At that time he had no idea of the details of the disease. The organism responsible for cholera would not be discovered for a quarter of a century, but that did not prevent this courageous and logical physician from analyzing the situation and taking action. His response was to do more than simply *treat* the diarrhea that cholera created; he removed the source and saved many lives. He did not wait the quarter of a century until a fuller understanding of the disease began to unfold. This is classical prevention. It's also of interest that the inconvenienced public failed to appreciate his action and civic leaders actively opposed him. Yet time and history proved him to be correct. We may have a similar opportunity today. It is not necessary to know all the fine details about the cause of breast cancer to take appropriate and effective action.

The German philosopher Immanuel Kant, wrote: "It is often necessary to make a decision on the basis of knowledge sufficient for action, but insufficient to satisfy the intellect." In the case of breast cancer and diet, I feel that the knowledge *is* sufficient to satisfy the intellect and form the basis for action. We need only to recognize the cause or causes, and remove them.

## Current Research and Treatment Trends

Research and treatment fads, as well as hopes and accomplishments, have been with us for years. Some of them have been of great importance and they are often of interest, but none has come close to solving the problem of breast cancer. Remember the search for the virus responsible for breast cancer? *Monoclonal antibodies* were the talk of the late 1970s and 1980s. More recently, genetic research and immunology have dominated the scientific scene. For years our researchers have sorted through thousands of compounds for effective, relatively nontoxic chemotherapeutic agents. To date we have only a handful and they are terribly toxic. These technologies are massive enterprises. The search for this kind of cure is expensive, glamorous, and headline grabbing, but it has also been remarkably ineffective in controlling breast cancer.

In my opinion, the most important new findings in breast cancer research have nothing to do with early diagnosis, mammography, surgical treatment, chemotherapy, radiation therapy, hormone therapy, genetic research, or any other high-tech modern developments. The most important development is the knowledge that women now have a means to prevent breast cancer from developing in the first place. Earliest possible detection of breast cancer is of undoubted value, but it is far preferable to avoid the problem.

## Diet Can Reduce Risk

The restriction of dietary fats and oils, accompanied by an increase in dietary fiber and other health-supporting foods, when practiced over the lifetime of an American woman will substantially reduce the probability of breast cancer taking her life. Note that these words are carefully chosen. I am not claiming that breast cancer can be totally eradicated, nor that all deaths from breast cancer are avoidable. But the totality of evidence supports the strong probability that breast cancer would be greatly reduced among women who decreased their fat intake to 15 percent of calories or less.

In order to be the powerful deterrent I am claiming them to be, these lifestyle changes should ideally start early in life, preferably before or during puberty. Does this mean that adults are out of luck, and that making lifestyle changes after puberty is too late? Not at all. The latest information shows that this plan can have positive health effects at any time, and there is very recent evidence that it can prolong the lives of women already diagnosed with breast cancer. Although changes made late in life will be less effective than changes made very early, *they are still worth making*. Some investigators in this field even think that postmenopausal women are more responsive to dietary influences than younger women.

Early detection of breast cancer is regarded as our best defense against that disease. I agree with all efforts that lead to the earliest possible discovery of disease, but it often is not enough. Let's look at an important reason why "early detection" so often fails. It takes a starting breast cancer, on average, about thirty cell divisions to reach a size where even the most sensitive detection methods can find the resulting tumor mass. Each of these divisions takes a specified amount of time. This is usually 110 days on average (the range is from 25 to 200 days). That means that many breast tumors have been developing for as long as *nine* years before they are first detectable! There are billions of cells in such a tumor when the earliest detection can be brought to bear. Even the rare, rapidly growing tumor usually takes more than two years to become detectable, and the slowest can take sixteen or more years. This slow growth affords the tumor ample time to spread to other parts of the body before it can be detected. This is a key to understanding the frequent failure of our early-detection efforts in breast cancer. It is the way-ward clumps of spreading cells (metastases) that cause death. The original breast cancer, growing in the breast itself, is almost never responsible for the death of a patient.

## The Prevention Message

Where do the doctors stand on this issue? It is safe to say that when most American doctors consider breast cancer, they are almost totally absorbed with detection and treat-ment. They seem to have very little interest in furthering any program of prevention. Our huge medical and surgical lit-erature concerning breast cancer clearly reflects this strong bias. Virtually all of the massive research output on the sub-ject of breast cancer has focused on treatment, detection, or basic biology. Only recently has there been even slight inter-est in the area of prevention—chiefly, by a pitifully small handful of doctors, maverick nutritionists, and the press—and some groups seem curiously intent on throwing cold wa-ter on all prevention efforts.

## Why Doctors Don't Know About Prevention

Why would well-trained and well-motivated doctors by-pass the vital issue of diet and prevention? Some of the rea-sons may be the following:

- Doctors were never trained to teach prevention.
- Most doctors are simply not aware of the research data.

• Professors and teachers did not impress upon them the importance of nutrition and prevention during their medical school years.

• Doctors prefer "high-tech" tools such as lasers, radiation therapy, complex surgical interventions, and chemotherapy.

• An interest in prevention is not consistent with the self-image of some physicians. They see themselves as the masters of complex, high-technology therapies.

• It's difficult for physicians to advocate a lifestyle that they do not personally follow.

• Some doctors feel that the teaching of nutrition is trivial or tedious work best left to paramedical professionals and nutritionists.

• Medical insurance usually will not pay doctors to teach lifestyle changes. At this time there is little profit in prevention. There is a faint possibility that this may change in the future, as it has in cardiac disease.

• Patients themselves are often reluctant to make changes in a lifestyle that they have selected because they prefer it. And doctors do not enjoy "fighting" with their patients to accomplish those changes.

Change can be difficult. A woman selects her diet because, as one of my patients told me, "I like it, I can afford it, and doctor, it's none of your business. What I do with my knife and fork is personal!" Some breast cancer experts call serious dietary change "culturally unacceptable." I think *breast cancer* is culturally unacceptable, and that promoting healthy eating plans should not only be highly culturally acceptable but critically necessary. Women should be given the information and the power to change their lives if they choose to do so. Many of my patients find a health-supporting diet to be not only feasible, but pleasurable. Deborah Bowen, a psychologist at the Fred Hutchinson Cancer Research Center in Seattle, studied 650 women for five years after they participated in a program of fat reduction where total fat calories were reduced from 37 to 23 percent. Eighty-two percent of the group continue to have success, and in the process experience less anxiety and depression as well as increased vigor and positive feelings.[23]

## What Would Be Absolute Proof for the Dietary Theory?

I am often challenged by colleagues who say: "You don't have absolute proof, so why should we burden our patients with this information? When you have ironclad proof, let's talk."

Absolute ironclad proof would require an absolutely perfect study. In the real world, this type of a study is impossible. For such a theoretically perfect study, we would need two very large and perfectly matched groups of female children with identical height, weight, health and family histories, environment, behavioral patterns, and activities. The only variable would be a wide difference in the percentage of dietary fat and fiber, which would be randomly assigned to the participants. Our ideal study would then be "put on ice" with the participants following the strict dietary guidelines for *fifty to sixty years* to allow the incidence of breast cancer in each group to become fully evident! Anything less than this clearly impossible study is open to at least some question.

Compared with our description of the "perfect" study of breast cancer causation, the Harvard Nurses' Study to be discussed later was nothing more than a mail survey of a high-risk group. And yet it was presented nationwide, and even internationally, as scientific truth. Many women took that report as a green light signaling them to eat whatever they wished, at least in reference to breast cancer risk. Many medical professionals viewed the study's findings on diet and breast cancer as definitive. It is impossible to imagine the extent of the disservice this study has done, because persuasive evidence exists that dietary fat does in fact increase breast cancer risk.

After many years of cancellations, false starts, political interferences, and redesigns, the National Institutes of Health has finally launched a $650-million fifteen-year study of more than 160,000 women to evaluate a variety of possible causes of breast cancer, including dietary fat. If you're willing to wait for fifteen or more years, hang on for the results. I'm not. We need information that we can act on now, even if it's not "definitive."

If the NIH study isn't well designed and properly executed, *it* won't be definitive either. My fear is that this study will serve as a justification for more than another decade of inaction while we wait for the results. In my experience as a breast cancer professional, delay is a particularly deadly form of denial.

# 4

## *Whom Can You Trust?*

*T*he intelligent woman who wants good health information today is inundated with strident but conflicting messages. One expert says that cholesterol is
all-important, while the next expert (from an equally prestigious university) will say that cholesterol is only a peripheral
issue. One year the word is that margarine is a health food,
and the next year it's said to be a near poison. Whom should
a woman believe? When it comes to breast cancer, our average American woman is finally getting the message that
diet, and particularly fat, *is* of great importance. Yet when
respected researchers from a top university say that fat is of
no importance whatever, whom should she trust? On matters
as important as her personal health and survival, she should
chiefly trust just one person. *She should trust herself.*

   I know what you're thinking. "But I don't know enough
about a subject as complicated as breast cancer to make such
important decisions!" You don't have to, any more than you
have to know how to design a house when you engage an
architect, or how to repair a car when you deal with an automobile repair agency. You are only required to be a knowl-
edgeable consumer. There is no substitute for shopping

around, learning the various viewpoints and strategies, and then using your own common sense and judgment. The following principles will help you to evaluate conflicting advice given to you.

• **Principle Number 1: It is better to prevent a disease than to treat it.**

This proposition is self-evident and requires no serious exposition. Yet, as stated so many times in this book, the medical establishment seems to have a very hard time in promoting prevention.

• **Principle Number 2: Women are biologically the same no matter where in the world they live.**

One of the great impediments to an understanding of breast cancer has been the refusal of medical and academic authorities to accept the pattern of disease in another country as representing a true response to the environment. They prefer to think of those differences as being genetic in origin. Breast cancer is chiefly an environmental disease. Otherwise, there is no reason why country of birth should be a risk factor for breast cancer. Why should a woman born in Scotland have a risk for development of breast cancer many times that of a similar appearing woman who was born in Poland? Why should a black woman born in America have a risk of breast cancer twenty times greater than a similar woman born in Kenya? *Why should place of birth be a risk factor for breast cancer?* Migration studies strongly suggest that the origins of breast cancer are chiefly environmental, not genetic. And if the environment is the major factor in the development of breast cancer, it can be modified. It is virtually certain that the strongest influence in the environment is nutrition. Nutrition, therefore, is the key to breast cancer prevention.

- **Principle Number 3: If breast cancer is largely an environmental disease, it can often be prevented.**

This is the essence of the entire breast cancer question. If breast cancer simply strikes a woman with no pattern or reason, then an attitude of waiting and doing what is possible with early detection and treatment makes sense. However, if the numbers of patients with this disease can be diminished (prevented) by dietary and lifestyle changes, then early detection *alone* would be an exceptionally unwise course.

My questions to the people who do not believe that breast cancer is caused, at least partially, by factors external to a woman's genetics are these: Why is it that the countries with the lowest per capita consumption of fat invariably have low levels of breast cancer? Why is it that the countries with the highest levels of fat intake invariably have the highest levels of breast cancer? Further, why is it that women from the low-breast-cancer-incidence countries who move to the high-incidence-breast-cancer countries (and adopt the dietary habits of the new country) develop breast cancer at the level of the high-incidence country? Why does their risk increase? What happens following their move?

I recently posed these questions to a distinguished panel of experts at an international breast cancer conference. Here's a synopsis of their vague and diversionary responses: "I don't think the fat theory is valid; the studies are in conflict," said one. Another said: "We need more studies." (This is the eternal cry of the researcher.) Response number three was: "Women just won't eat that way!" How did these male experts feel that they could speak for the women of America? What mandate did they have? What research and polling have they done on that subject? All sincere scientific efforts to determine whether women are able to follow a truly low-fat diet have been met with remarkable success. These are called feasibility studies, and there are many of them. The final comment from the panel was: "Yes, there may be something to prevention and we are hoping to start a chemo-prevention trial with tamoxifen." These doctors seem to believe that placing women on a powerful medication costing up to $100 per month is preferable to changing the food they eat. We're back to the establishment "a pill for every ill" concept. Not one of the experts directly answered the questions.

Can you imagine the financial impact of *millions* of women swallowing two pills each day in the hope that these pills will allow them to continue eating the 35 to 40 percent fat standard American diet and escape breast cancer? This is *very big business.* Is it possible that huge profits may be getting in the way of more sober scientific considerations? An extensive discussion of the informed consent issue was presented in the November, 1992, *Science News.* Noting that the drug can induce cancer and fatal blood clots, they wonder if volunteers for the study are sufficiently informed of the risks. I place many of my breast cancer patients on tamoxifen, it is an excellent drug *when properly used in the treatment of cancer,* especially for postmenopausal women with estrogen receptor positive tumors. However, that is *not the same* as placing healthy people on the same regimen. Several of my patients have been forced to discontinue their tamoxifen by night sweats so severe that their bedclothes are soaked and they are unable to rest. Others have had severe depression. An excess of uterine cancer has been observed. There are other potential problems including eye diseases, damage to the fetus should a premenopausal women become pregnant, development of a drug-resistant and aggressive breast tumor, and liver tumors. Italian investigators are sufficiently concerned about the uterine cancer issue that they are testing the drug only in women who have had hysterectomies. In short, all medicines pose risk. Is this a reasonable and ethical study? Are there more rational and economically preferable alternatives? Will the participants in the study be given all of the facts relevant to the risks, as well as the advantages? I can think of no precedent for this type of study in American medicine and find it a bad idea. Breast cancer is not caused by a tamoxifen deficiency.

• **Principle Number 4: Base your thinking on the totality of evidence, not on a single study.**

It is possible to defend almost any viewpoint with fragments of evidence selectively culled from the scientific literature. This tactic is called *selective quotation* and I have tried not to be guilty of it in this book. The *totality* of the credible evidence should be the basis of your evaluation. Remember, though, that there have been times when the body of scientific literature and all involved experts were entirely wrong. A theory should have a logical and reasonable basis. It also should work when applied to "real world" problems. When you hold our current medical thinking about breast cancer to these standards, it does not fare well.

When you test the breast cancer/dietary fat theory in this manner, it proves to be accurate and correct. *No other theory matches the facts so well.* Learn the facts and then make your own decisions concerning breast cancer prevention. Empower yourself.

# 5

# The Diet Connection: The Evidence

*I*t is not my intention to dismiss scientific research. In fact, the breast cancer story is clearly told by evidence gathered from around the world by scientific researchers. Let's draw together the global evidence available to us—studies that have been largely ignored by our own medical establishment—and summarize the evidence concerning the causes of breast cancer.

## Human Population Studies

*Epidemiology* is one of the oldest and most important medical disciplines. It compares populations, not individuals, to learn what causes one group to fall prey to a disease and another to escape it. It also searches for common characteristics among persons who contract specific diseases. Over the years, lessons learned from epidemiology have saved thousands of lives. This may be the best single tool available to scientists searching for the causes of breast cancer.

Epidemiology shows us without a doubt that women in the United States, the United Kingdom, Canada, Australia, and Northern Europe have a breast cancer incidence five or even six times higher than women from Asian and African countries. The contrast between the very highest and the very lowest countries is even greater. *In countries with low breast cancer incidence there is low intake of dietary fat. In countries with high levels of breast cancer there is high intake of fat.* This relationship of high-fat diets to high breast cancer rates is strikingly consistent in all countries studied. *There are no exceptions.* This information alone should be enough to cause a thoughtful woman to markedly reduce her dietary fat intake.

The dietary differences observed among the world's countries are substantial, and their effect on individuals starts in infancy. If the environmental and dietary theory is correct, there should be clear differences among women in different countries. The evidence shows that these differences do exist. (It should also be noted that there is an unavoidable, baseline level of breast cancer in every country studied, even in those with the very lowest levels of fat intake and the very lowest breast cancer incidence.) Breast cancer rates are approximately *twelve times greater, or even twenty-five times greater* in some countries where high-fat diets are the norm when compared with those where fat consumption is low.

## Migration Studies

*Epidemiologic studies* do not remove the possibility that genetic differences might account for the differing rates, but migration studies do. *Migration studies* show that women who move from areas with a low incidence of breast cancer (such as Japan) to less "protected" areas (such as the United States) will have an increased rate of breast cancer. The rate of breast cancer among their daughters is even higher than that of their mothers, and is little different from any other women in the adopted country. All of the above is seen only in those women who adapt to the dietary habits of their new country. The time period required for the increase in breast cancer incidence can be as short as eight to ten years. These migration studies are critically important as they strongly indicate that the "protection" conferred on women in countries with low rates of breast cancer is *environmental*, not genetic.

In all there have been more than eleven migration studies. For example, two have tracked Italian women who migrated to Australia and Polish women who came to the United States. In each case, women who moved to an area of higher breast cancer incidence have developed more breast cancer. Also, in every case cited, the higher breast cancer rate followed a higher dietary fat intake. Other migration studies included Taiwanese women coming to the United States, Yemenites to Israel, Ethiopians to Israel, Parsee women to India, and currently, Filipina women to California.

Even within-country migrations have shown higher levels of breast cancer, but only if the fat intake is increased. These studies have taken place in Italy[24, 25] where there is a dramatic difference in breast cancer deaths in the south (19.1 deaths per 100,000 population) compared with the north (26.1 deaths per 100,000). The United States rate is 27.1 per 100,000 and our meat intake is two times greater than that of southern Italy. Women who migrate from the Asian Russian republics to the European Russian republics also experience an increase in their breast cancer rates as they accommodate to the food and living conditions in the more Westernized areas.

Although it does not deal with a current migration, a most intriguing study compares African-American women with women living in Africa. Their initial migration, although involuntary, took place well over a hundred and fifty years ago. Such research is difficult to conduct because of the relative scarcity of data from Africa. However, one 1976

# International Breast Cancer Death Rates Related to Fat Intake

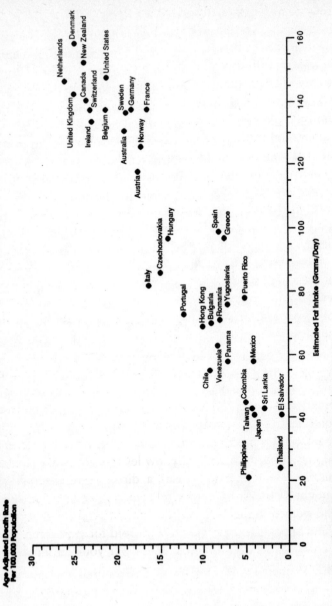

Adapted from Carroll, K.K Cancer Research vol. 35:3374 - 3383. 1975

study reported the African breast cancer rate as being one third that of Western women. A 1992 study from Kenya puts the incidence of breast cancer in that country at an astonishingly low 1.08 cases per 100,000 women![26] This is nearly twentyfold less than the U.S. average. Medical authorities who have worked in both areas have long had the strong clinical impression that the difference is dramatic. Far greater numbers of African-American women die of breast cancer than African women. This further supports the diet/cancer connection. Another poorly studied part of the world with a similar lifestyle is New Guinea, which has a very low reporting rate of 2.7 cases per 100,000 women.[27] Again, this is an area where extremely low fat levels exist in the local diet.

In every one of these studies, a higher fat and lower fiber diet resulted in a loss of what was previously thought to be genetic protection. Higher levels of breast cancer invariably followed. Migration studies alone are sufficient to convince me of the importance of lifestyle change.

One of the lowest levels of breast cancer recorded occurs in a province in China where fat ingestion is a remarkably low 6 percent of calories. The consistency in these studies is remarkable—and the correlation with dietary fat always holds true. Dr. T. Colin Campbell found the range of fat intake among Chinese women to be from 6 to 24 percent of calories.[28] This is a strikingly low level of fat intake. Despite this, he found that there was a direct relationship to the amount of breast cancer found *even within that low range*. The women in the 24-percent counties had the highest rates. There appears to be no lower threshold for protection when it comes to fat consumption. The lower your fat intake, the more protection you receive.

## Time-Trend Studies

*Time-trend studies* examine the relationship between changes over time in consumption of fat or other foods and the rates of breast cancer in one particular population. The Japanese experience is the most dramatic in this regard; sharp increases in breast cancer followed the increase of fat in the Japanese diet since World War II. In 1950, fat intake was an exceptionally low 7.5 percent of all calories; by 1955, it increased to 9 percent of all calories—still remarkably low for a technologically advanced society. By the 1970s, fat intake had increased to 18 percent. Now, as the Japanese are becoming more Westernized, the level is currently 28 percent of total calories and still rising. Among American exports to Japan are beef and tobacco as well as fast-food franchises. Japanese dairy, meat, egg, and chicken consumption has increased eightfold. Dairy products, almost unavailable before World War II, are now used at nearly twenty times the prewar rates.[29] Those dairy products were introduced into the Japanese school lunch program by the occupying U.S. authorities in 1946. At the same time that the Japanese have been increasing these foodstuffs, they have been radically decreasing their consumption of beta-carotenes and even rice.[30]

The Japanese have quadrupled their fat consumption over a thirty-year period with intake approaching eighty-five grams per capita by the middle 1980s.[31] If limiting consumption of these foods were as important as I have alleged, the breast cancer rates in Japan should have decisively increased since the end of World War II. They have. Japanese breast cancer incidence rose 58 percent between 1975 and 1985 alone. The Japanese example is particularly instructive for Americans, because the United States and Japan are nearly equivalent in industrial development, education, medical care, and medical record keeping. Even the benign breast lumps biopsied in Japan are showing an increase in atypia, or tendency toward malignancy.[32]

In the late 1960s, I spent several fascinating months as a volunteer surgeon in South Vietnam working in the civilian hospitals. I never saw a case of breast cancer. I am now told that in all of Vietnam, the incidence of breast cancer is rapidly rising and is approaching 60 percent of the United States' incidence. Breast cancer is now the leading cause of cancer mortality among women in North Vietnam.[33]

What about our dietary changes in the United States? Use of fats and oils has increased by 23 percent since 1965. Most of these increases are in edible oils (cooking, salad, and vegetable), the consumption of which has increased by a whopping 77 percent. Another source lists this figure at a 65 percent increase in polyunsaturated fat. Other changes include a 10 percent increase in poultry, fish, and shellfish and a drop in red meat consumption. In the same period, the use of eggs is down 18 percent; whole milk usage is down 48 percent; low-fat milk, yogurt, and cheese are all up more than 100 percent. While our current fat intake is estimated at 34 to 37 percent of all calories (down from 42 percent), it is still **far** too high. Despite this, some authorities feel that there has not been a decrease in total fat consumption. Using a method called *per capita disappearance data*, one notices that there has been an overall 18-percent *increase* in total fat consumed in the United States between 1960 and 1985.[34]

A much safer level of total fat ingestion is 15 to 20 percent of calories. The ideal for breast cancer prevention would be 10 percent of total calories as fat—or even a lower level, as we learned in the Cornell-China study.

Despite a debated drop in fat intake, the breast cancer rates are still increasing. Is this a delayed response to the previous increases or is there another reason?

In my opinion, the data support a link between increased use of vegetable oils and hydrogenated fats with the increase in breast cancer rates. In the 1960s, when the association between saturated fat, cholesterol, and heart disease was established, we radically increased our intake of vegetable oils and hydrogenated fats in an attempt to escape coronary artery disease while maintaining our dietary preferences. We responded by embracing the "good oils" and "noncholesterol" products. Instead of cutting the use of fats overall, Americans were encouraged to increase their use of "good" fats in the mistaken belief that they were harmless or even beneficial. As a result, the average American now ingests over twenty-one pounds of all oils each year! I believe that this unprecedented change in human nutrition has had a massive negative impact on our health. The dramatic increase in consumption of oils and especially the hydrogenated fats is not even mentioned in much of the published research on this subject. It appears that we have partially protected our hearts by reducing the saturated fats in our diet, but have caused increases in breast, prostate, and colon cancers.

In a number of animal studies, polyunsaturated fats are seen to be more effective promoters of breast cancer than saturated fats, although *total* fat intake remains the main determinant. Other researchers feel that human breast cancer increase is due to pesticides, radiation from exposure to mammography, electromagnetic fields, stress, or even less likely possibilities such as hair dye, iron overload in the diet, and even excessive exposure to light during nighttime hours. I am not convinced by such data, but I remain open to new and verifiable information.

Some people confuse polyunsaturated fats with the essential fatty acids our bodies require for optimal health. They are not the same. Many polyunsaturated fatty acids are not essential and may be harmful. (The human body cannot manufacture essential fatty acids; they must come from outside food sources.) Seeds and leafy plants are the principle sources of both of the prime essential fatty acids (EFAs). Plankton, or marine plant life, is at the base of the marine food chain enriching fish with another useful fat group, the omega-3 acids. The omega-3 and omega-6 are organic chemistry designations. The lower numbers are generally the most beneficial. The omega-3 fats have anticlotting properties that interfere with factors that promote heart attacks. These fats are also involved with a class of compounds called prostaglandins that have anti-inflammatory effects.

Unlike an automobile engine, the human body does not run well on oils. Ask yourself this question: Were processed, concentrated oils available to our ancestors 60,000 years ago? Of course not; oils are artificial, man-made foods. The oil content in plant foods, *as grown*, is ideal. That content usually ranges from 2 to 6 percent of total calories. The fats that we don't need are the refined or hydrogenated fats. The process of refining involves heat, chemical solvents, caustics, bleach, deodorizers, and exposure to oxygen. *The resultant oils resemble chemicals more than food* and they are usually packaged in clear containers that allow even further oxidation damage and deterioration from exposure to light. Our bodies are not designed to digest and metabolize chemicals; they are designed to digest food exactly as those foods are found in nature.

If you're looking for a "good" oil, olive oil is probably the least dangerous but it is still not recommended in large quantities as a "health food." It is over 80 percent monounsaturated fat with about 10 percent saturated fat. Use it sparingly. The type of fat you eat is important. For example, omega-3 oils found in fish are less carcinogenic than the fats found in beef. There is evidence from Norway that women eating a greater proportion of fish than beef have reduced rates of breast cancer. Even the method of preparation seems to be important. In the Norwegian studies, poached fish was more protective than fish prepared in other ways. The relative risk for women who ate meat dinners five times or more per week was 1.8 (nearly two times "normal"). The risk for the poached fish eaters was only 0.7. This was the conclusion of a fourteen-year study of over 14,000 women reported in the *International Journal of Cancer* in 1990.[35]

## Analytic Epidemiology

*Analytic epidemiology* is a term for studies based on comparisons of individuals or groups of individuals *within* a society. These studies generally support the diet/breast cancer link but suffer from a variety of weaknesses. It is generally among these studies that the conflicting and confusing results are found. The chief reasons for this are high levels of fat ingestion for the entire group, inaccurate methods of assessing fat intake, and study periods that are too brief. The studies can be designed to include groups already diagnosed with breast cancer (*case-control* studies) or those free of the disease to see who develops breast cancer (*cohort* studies).

An example of the latter is the 1987 Harvard Nurses' Health Study referred to in Chapter 3. Here, a drop in the percentage of fat intake from 44 to 32 percent had minimal effect. Critics of the dietary fat/breast cancer hypothesis claimed that the fat reduction had no effect, and that fat therefore had nothing to do with breast cancer. But in this study design, the reduction in fat intake was simply too small, the range too narrow, and the time too short to allow for a meaningful effect. Also lacking was a study group with a 15 to 20 percent fat diet. We know from our epidemiological studies that a fat intake of *20 percent of calories or less* is needed for protection against breast cancer.

## Animal Studies

Animal studies have always been extremely important in cancer research. All mammals have a remarkable underlying unity of molecular biological behavior. There is very little difference between the way animal and human breast tissues respond to dietary factors. Here are some of the key findings from animal studies:

• For more than seventy-five years, researchers have consistently found that an increase in dietary fat causes an increase in the spontaneous growth of breast cancers in those animals prone to develop breast cancers. The first American researcher to note this was Kanematsu Sugiura at what later became the Sloan-Kettering Institute in New York. The year? 1917![36]

• Tumor growth increases when high levels of fat are given (even after spontaneous initiation of breast cancer). The conclusion: *dietary fat is a promoting agent for breast cancer growth in animals.*

• Dietary fat and total caloric intake (with its resulting obesity) seem to have separate and independent tumor-enhancing effects, although each can act alone to increase breast cancer growth.

• Increases in dietary fiber protect against breast cancer, even in animals.

• When the animal's ovaries are removed, thus eliminating nearly all estrogen, the addition of fat is **still** able to weakly increase the incidence of breast cancer.

In a 1992 study, human breast cancer cells were implanted in a strain of hairless mice without thymus glands (these so-called nude, athymic mice have greatly reduced immunity). Groups of such mice were given diets containing differing amounts of corn oil (5 percent and 23 percent). These human tumors grew and spread more rapidly in the group given the high-corn-oil diet.[37]

In another study, mice were given breast cancer by the injection of breast cancer cells intravenously. They were then given diets enriched in cruciferous vegetables (cabbage and collards). This resulted in a reduced spread of cancer. These results support the contention that diets high in cruciferous vegetables may be beneficial in cancer prevention.[38]

In a study comparing the effect of different fats, identical groups of mice grafted with human breast cancer cells were fed lard, corn oil, and fish oil. The fish oil group had the slowest rate of tumor growth when compared with the other two groups.[39]

Yet another study in Japan showed that it was possible to stimulate mammary tumor growth in rats with a high-fat diet and then to "switch it off" with a change to a low-fat diet.[40]

The results of animal experimentation strongly support the link between high-fat diets and breast cancer.

## The Test of Biological Plausibility

Does the dietary theory have a reasonable and probable biologic basis? This is a fundamental scientific question, and the answer is yes for a number of reasons:

• We know that breast cancer is a *hormone-dependent* disease. It almost never develops in the absence of estrogen.
• It has been demonstrated that dietary fat intake closely relates to estrogen levels in a woman's body. Increasing dietary fat increases the estrogen levels, while decreasing the fat decreases those levels. That is how fat "feeds" or promotes breast cancer.

- Fat has carcinogenic or cancer-promoting effects.

- Metabolic carcinogens (cancer-causing compounds) can result from a high-fat diet.

- Studies have shown that DNA repair is impaired by high-fat diets. Researchers at Wayne State University in Detroit randomly assigned high-risk women to one of two groups. One group ate their usual diet (35 to 40 percent of calories as fat) and the other group was taught to eat a diet with only 15 calories from fat. Analysis of oxidation damage to the DNA of the participants' red blood cells showed that the damage to the DNA was reduced by two-thirds in the low-fat intervention group.[41]

- Dietary fat has been shown to act as a promoting factor for the growth of breast cancer.

- Dietary fat can suppress the immune system. Natural "killer" cells are a key part of the body's ability to destroy cancer cells. These killer cells are white blood cells that seek out malignant cells and bacteria. The activity of these killer cells is markedly increased on low-fat diets. The opposite is true with high-fat diets, in which the fats appear to inhibit the immune system.[42, 43, 44, 45] Beta-carotenes also increase the activity of natural killer cells as well as other beneficial cells called T-helper cells that originate in the thymus gland.[46]

- Dietary fat promotes a variety of other cancers. Colon cancer, prostate cancer, uterine cancer, ovarian cancer, pancreatic cancer, and even lung cancer have all been associated with increased levels of dietary fat.

- High-fat diets alter the type of bacteria that colonize the large intestine, favoring a type (anaerobic bacteria) that causes a breakdown of estrogen complexes. This results in greater reabsorption of estrogen and higher blood levels of the hormone. It is normal to eliminate excess estrogen in the stool. Estrogen levels in the stool are decidedly lower in meat-eating women compared with strict vegetarian women. The estrogen is reabsorbed in the blood of the meat eaters.

- High-fat diets are almost always low-fiber diets. And because low-fiber diets increase hormone levels, their effect in facilitating breast cancer is additive.

• The opposite is also true. Increases in dietary fiber decrease hormone levels because of changes in absorption of digestive bile salts and increased excretion of hormones from the intestine.

• Certain types of dietary fats damage the outer lining of bodily cells (the plasma membranes) as well as the DNA in the inner portion or nucleus of the cells. These critical injuries can increase the incidence of cancer.

The dietary fat/cancer link is logical, plausible, and supported by the data. It would be illogical to suppose that a high-fat diet would not cause an increase in breast cancer.

## The Evolutionary Model

Speaking in geological time, it was only recently that our hunter-gatherer ancestors lived on wild foods from the land, and to a lesser extent from rivers, lakes, and seas. During that time period the physiology of today's women developed, adapting precisely to those wild foods. Our bodies are *still* designed for those living conditions; there has been no significant change. Our genetic heritage is virtually the same as it was many millions of years ago. Our physiology and biochemistry are attuned to the conditions of life that existed in the Paleolithic era. The profound differences between the environment of ancient women and the environment of today's women is possibly the single most important key to the breast cancer riddle.

This observation has been called the *discordance hypothesis*. We are living in discord with our true nature. The fat intake of our Paleolithic ancestors is estimated to have been less than half our current intake. In addition to that, the fat they ate was higher in polyunsaturated than saturated fat, the reverse of our modern pattern. Their food supply was also far richer in dietary fiber.[47]

In an August 1993 *Scientific American* article entitled "Diet and Primate Evolution," Katharine Milton, a professor of anthropology at the University of California, Berkeley, says the following: "Foods eaten by humans today, especially those consumed in industrially advanced nations, bear little resemblance to the plant-based diets anthropoids have favored since their emergence. Such findings lend support to the suspicion that many health problems common in technologically advanced nations may result, at least in part, from a mismatch between the diets we now eat and those to which our bodies became adapted over millions of years." Milton's studies led her to conclude that ancient humans became omnivores only after their plant-food supplies became inadequate through competition from other animals. She feels that the practice of adding meat to the previously vegetarian diet created the division of labor between members of the group, the development of social cooperation, and the development of larger brains. However, the digestive processes of humans did not change. She continues: "Although the practice of adding some amount of meat to the regular daily intake became a pivotal force in the emergence of modern humans, this behavior does not mean that people today are biologically suited to the virtually fiber-free diet many of us now consume. In fact, in its general form, our digestive tract does not seem to be greatly modified from that of the common ancestor apes and humans, which was undoubtedly a strongly herbivorous animal."

The Agricultural Revolution occurred only 8,000 to 12,000 years ago, initiating gradual shifts away from natural foods, which resulted in progressive damage to human health. The Industrial Revolution greatly accelerated these damaging changes. There have been only a few generations of humans since then—clearly not a sufficient number to permit adaptation. Moreover, the creation of food surpluses and high-fat diets for entire societies over only the last hundred years has been unprecedented in human history.

These changes have been accompanied by a startling increase in cancer and degenerative diseases.[48] We have further worsened our nutritional environment by altering the domestic animals whose bodies we eat. We have done this through selective breeding and by the administration of hormones, antibiotics, and artificially fattening foods in order to create the obese, ill creatures whose flesh we "prefer."

Why do we gravitate toward fatty foods? Can we trust our instincts? Many of my patients tell me that their bodies "need" beef or cheese. They have cravings they interpret as the "wisdom of the body" urging them to do the right thing. This is a naive notion. When left to their own devices with unlimited access to any type of food, rats do exactly the same thing humans have done in America; *they select a diet rich in fat*. A researcher named Morris H. Ross investigated this in 1974, reporting his findings in *Nature*. He observed that rats allowed to select their own food grew rapidly, became larger, and matured sexually sooner than other animals on a variety of other dietary regimens. But these free-eating rats also developed more cancers and died earlier than the others. Ross concluded that the instinctive behavior of the animals was the result of "species survival instincts" formed in prehistoric times to protect against starvation and ensure the survival of the breed. The fatty food does not assure health, but merely acts as a concentrated source of calories and a defense against death from starvation. Other, more recent theories hold that when humans live sedentary lives, their bodies crave calorically dense, or rich and fatty, foods. Whatever the reason for our fatal attraction to fatty foods, it is *not* the body's attempt to insure good health.

Can Ross's findings offer an insight into our own self-destructive behaviors? These survival instincts were formed during the evolutionary process to protect us from starvation and therefore have no relevance to the realities of today's world for American women and men. There may be other, even less well-understood aspects of "instinctive" tastes. Neuroscience is a relatively new field of medical research. Researchers in this field claim that, in rats, a brain protein called galanin drives the animal's craving for fatty foods. As you would expect, scientists are working on a drug to block the action of galanin. What about the craving that some experience for tobacco, for alcohol, for heroin and cocaine? Clearly there are substances that are not good for us but that can grip us, either from an instinctive drive (fat to avoid starvation) or from a neurochemical pleasure center (tobacco, cocaine, and other drugs). Our dietary preferences and pleasures are not erratic, random choices. They represent previous necessities in human history. However, those guidelines from our evolutionary past can betray us in the present.

Meat samples from wild animals are rich in essential polyunsaturated fatty acids and very low in saturated, storage fat. By contrast, the modern "marbled" beef prized by today's gourmets is infiltrated by fat that is largely of the dangerous, saturated type. In many pieces of "choice" beef, the fat accounts for more than 60 percent of total calories. Fat in wild land animals is never more than 4 percent by weight. Our Paleolithic ancestors would have found it impossible to follow a high-fat diet even if they had chosen to! Today we seem to raise our feedlot animals more for fat than for protein. Even our much-heralded chicken has become far fatter in the past few decades of factory farming. Chicken breast without skin is 19-percent fat. Thighs without skin can be as high as 47-percent fat. The fat content of chicken has tripled in the last twenty-five years. Many of the patients who come to my office with fat-related illnesses, and with high cholesterol levels, all exclaim as if they had rehearsed it together: "But doctor, I can't understand it. I've cut out most red meat and I'm eating plenty of chicken and fish!"

Meat isn't the only culprit. Watch the oils, too. Our ancient ancestors had no access to concentrated, artificial, and man-made substances such as oils. It takes fourteen ears of corn to produce one tablespoon of corn oil. You wouldn't think of eating that amount of corn! Yet we casually eat food that contains several times that amount of oil in a single serving. *Our bodies are simply not designed to tolerate such amounts of oil.* Diets high in vegetable oils have been found to suppress the immune system and thus promote the growth and spread of cancer.[49]

It is also worth noting that chickens and cattle are very often fattened by adding estrogen to their feed. In Puerto Rico, Italy, and West Germany, there have been instances of severe hormonal poisoning of children from chicken, pork, veal, and milk unlawfully fattened or contaminated with estrogens. Menstrual periods, uterine enlargement, ovarian cysts, breast development, body hair, and premature puberty in girls as young as four years were traced to hormonally contaminated foods! In the United States, hormone levels are not as high, and yet from 30 to 90 percent of the chickens, 80 percent of veal calves and pigs, and 60 percent of the beef cattle raised for food are given hormones mixed with their feed. These additives are not always neutralized by cooking, and the ingested hormones can directly stimulate the breast tissue of women eating such food. Meat not only can be contaminated with bacteria, but can also be contaminated with hormones. Europeans have banned the import of American beef because of hormone contamination.

By and large, the diet followed by the majority of societies throughout the long span of human history has been of the health-supporting type that I am urging today's women to follow. Let's examine the dietary patterns of eight important societal groups. (The source of this material is chiefly the work of Will Durant, namely: *Our Oriental Heritage*, 1954; *The Life of Greece*, 1939; and *Caesar and Christ*, 1957).[50]

The Babylonians, nestled in the cradle of civilization thousands of years before Christ, produced a variety of grains, peas, beans, lentils, fruits, nuts, and the date palm. Goat milk and cheese, along with grapes and olives, supplemented the diet. Meat was rarely used and costly, but even the poorest families could afford an occasional fish. Wine made from dates and beer made from barley rounded out their menu.

Slightly to the north lived the Assyrians, whose famous capital, Ninevah, is known to Bible readers. Their fields yielded an abundance of wheat, barley, millet, and sesame. Also cultivated were olives, grapes, garlic, onions, lettuce, watercress, beets, turnips, radishes, cucumbers, and even licorice. Again, meat was rarely eaten except by the aristocracy. Except for fish taken from the Tigris River, this powerful warring nation was nearly vegetarian.

Throughout the long history of India, the majority of people have lived on a diet of rice, peas, lentils, millet, vegetables, and fruit. Meat, including fish and fowl, was eaten only by the rich or, in ancient times, by outcasts. Hindus made their cuisine more varied and interesting by the addition of spices including curry, ginger, cloves, cinnamon, and pepper.

Rice paddies and millet fields dominated the rural landscape of China. However, wheat and barley were also important grains. Added to these are a long list of legumes and vegetables, berries, and fruits. Perhaps the most important crop besides rice was the versatile soybean, from which the Chinese make soy milk and soy cheese. Cow's milk was almost nonexistent and eggs were not plentiful. Traditionally, rice, macaroni, vermicelli, vegetables, and small pieces of fish have made up the diet of the poor. The rich have always indulged their passion for duck.

The Japanese have always followed a simple diet consisting of rice, vegetables, seaweed, fruit, and small pieces of meat. Meat was a luxury afforded chiefly to the aristocracy and the military. One observer noted that "On a regimen of rice, a little fish and no meat, a Japanese man developed good lungs and tough muscles, and could run from fifty to eighty miles in twenty-four hours without distress; when he added meat he lost this capacity." Japanese acquaintance with beef is very recent, and the Gyokusenji Temple in Shimoda marks the spot where the first cow was killed in Japan for human consumption. The year was 1930. The chains around the memorial were a gift from the U.S. Navy. Where do you suppose the Japanese got the idea to start eating beef? We introduced milk into their school eating plans following World War II, and everyone knows about the current invasion of our fast-food franchises. One 1993 report described a new, American fast-food outlet opening every ninety minutes in Japan!

Even in their harsh mountainous land, the ancient Greeks were an especially vigorous people whose staple grain was barley. From barley they made porridge, flat breads, and cakes, often mixed with honey. Olive oil, figs, grapes, wine, goat cheese, beans, peas, cabbage, lentils, lettuce, onions, garlic, and many other condiments rounded out their everyday foods. Meat was rarely eaten, but fish, shark, and eels were common additions to the regular diet. Water was the normal drink, but diluted wine was available at every meal.

The diet of the ancient Romans was very similar to that of the Greeks. "Breakfast consisted of barley or wheat bread with honey, olives or cheese. Lunch and dinner were made up of grains, fruit, and vegetables. Diluted wine was served, but only the rich ate fish or meat. As the Roman empire began to decline, meals became exceptionally rich and long, with many courses of meats, game, and delicacies such as caviar, oyster, and anchovies."[51]

In Mexico the basic crop for over five thousand years has been corn. Even today, maize or corn is the most important single item in Mexico's diet. This grain together with beans, tomatoes, onions, peppers, and small amounts of meat has always been the standard Mexican meal. Mexican cuisine abounds in an array of fruits, berries, coffees, and assorted vegetables. Fish, chicken, beef, and eggs are rarely eaten in large quantities. The cow was unknown prior to the advent of the Spaniards. Until then, the largest animal eaten was a guinea pig–like creature. The extensive use of lard is also a recent addition.

In nearly all cultures, one of the grains has provided humans with a majority of their essential carbohydrate and protein. Throughout Asia, that grain continues to be rice. In Europe and North America, the favored grain has been wheat. In Mexico and Latin America, corn is the main foodstuff. In other parts of the world, the carbohydrate is millet, manioc, or taro. When people learned to prefer polished rice and wheat (thus removing much of the valuable fiber, minerals, and vitamins), they also began a pattern of poor food preparation that continues to haunt us today. Were it not for the many technological "advances" in mass production, canning, refrigeration, and freezing, Americans would not have easy access to so many of the "wrong" foods.

There are several groups that developed markedly unusual eating patterns. The Eskimos and the Masai are the two most often mentioned; their eating plans resulted in serious health problems. In each case arteriosclerosis resulted, but the Eskimos were also plagued with severe osteoporosis and the Masai with arthritis. These groups are mentioned only because they are often cited as "evidence" that fat is not harmful. Only factors such as the preponderance of omega-3 fats from fish-based foods for the Eskimos, and extreme exertion and excellent physical conditioning for the Masai, salvaged the situation.

We have sharply deviated from the wise path of our ancestors. Since they were virtually free from the diseases that now plague us, even when corrections are made for length of life, we must conclude that our present-day eating plan is tragically unhealthful.

## Genetics

I can't remember how many times I have heard doctors say, "Well, it doesn't matter *what* you do; it's all in your genes." Many of them seem to believe that heredity is the prime risk factor for breast cancer. I don't. More than 80 percent of our new patients with breast cancer have negative family histories for that disorder. The consensus of modern thought on the subject holds that breast cancer results from the combined action of many genes (unalterable) and the patient's environment (alterable). With this understanding we can see that breast cancer is not the result of a genetic accident or bad luck except in rare instances. It also affords us the comforting knowledge that we have a measure of control over this disease and are not simply passive victims. In most cases, breast cancer is the result of predictable biological responses to the way we live. Remember also the instructive twin studies that showed us that genetic tendencies are not all-powerful. The rare BRCA 1 gene is the notable exception, but it affects less than one half of one percent of American women.

There is a genetic component to nearly every disease. Breast cancer is no exception. What is inherited is a *susceptibility* to develop breast cancer, not the disease itself. It is often impossible to separate the effect of genetics from the effect of the learning how to live that takes place in the home—this is the *familial* factor. It is in the home that the child learns to eat from the example provided by family members. In the Danish adoption study discussed earlier, the family environment was five times more powerful than genetics in determining the probability of death from cancer. Breast cancer is, in the main, a *familial*, not a genetic disease.

To illustrate how this linkage may operate, Nomura, Henderson, and Lee carried out a unique study among Japanese-Americans living in Hawaii. Eighty-six Japanese men out of a total study group of 6,860 men were married to women who developed breast cancer. It was assumed that the men ate diets similar to those of their wives. It was then determined that these men ate more beef, meats, hot dogs, margarine, butter, and cheese than the other men. They also ate less Japanese food than the controls (men whose wives had not developed breast cancer). The authors concluded that certain American foods are important in the search for the dietary factors that cause breast cancer in women.[52]

Demonstrating the familial aspects of breast cancer, a study published in the *Journal of the American Medical Association*[53] informs us that a woman's risk of breast cancer is doubled if her mother had breast cancer diagnosed before age forty. However, it was less than doubled (relative risk=1.8) for all women whose mothers had breast cancer. The diagnosis of breast cancer in a woman's sister increases risk as well. For women with two or more sisters, if one was diagnosed with breast cancer, the risk for the uninvolved sisters was nearly two times greater (relative risk=1.9). Overall, within the large population studied (nearly 118,000 women), only 2.5 percent of breast cancer cases were attributed to a positive family history. I conclude that breast cancer is far more a familial disease than a genetic disease.

## The World War Evidence

What possible relationship can exist between two world wars and the incidence of breast cancer? Epidemiologists found, to their amazement, that the rates of nearly all cancers (as well as heart disease) fell during World War I[54] and remained relatively low for some years after![55] In Denmark, the Allied blockade during World War I caused shortages of food for their livestock. The Danish minister of health, Dr. Michael Hindhede, responded by ordering the killing of nearly all the livestock and the conversion of the arable land to the raising of food for the populace. This forced the people of Denmark to become instant and unwilling near vegetarians. But it also resulted in a *one-third reduction of the overall death rate from non–war-related diseases.*[56] This was a great surprise to those early investigators. Owing to the widespread lack of butter, milk, eggs, cheese, meat, lard, and other nutrients then thought to be essential for good health, they had been expecting to find an increase in disease.

The same association was discovered during and after World War II.[57] The scientific analysis and the data collection were much better than in the World War I study, and the conclusions far more reliable. Rates of heart disease and cancer did not return to the prewar levels until seven years following the conflict.[58] The diet forced on European populations by food shortages was based on grains and vegetables. It was extremely low in fat. Exercise levels increased as well. Believers in the stress theory of heart disease and cancer causation should note that the effects of the low-fat diet outweighed the effects of fear, anxiety, and stress.

Even now, in England and Scotland, researchers from the Cancer Research Campaign are observing a dip in breast cancer rates for women in their late fifties and sixties. Their most plausible explanation is that wartime shortages of meat and dairy products during the Second World War forced five or six years of a low-fat diet on those women and gave them a degree of protection during the highly critical developmental years surrounding puberty and menarche.

This finding parallels that of a similar Italian study by

Franco Berrino and Gemma Gatta from the renowned Milan Cancer Institute. They found that young women going through puberty in the southern part of Italy during World War II had a greatly reduced incidence of breast cancer compared to clearly matched women from the north of Italy, where food shortages were not so severe. The difference was over fivefold![59]

A third wartime study, this one again in Norway, described a reduction in breast cancer incidence in women experiencing adolescence during the World War II period of fat and calorie restriction.[60]

Other researchers have also postulated that a high-fat diet during puberty and adolescence increases the risk of breast cancer later in life.[61] There is remarkable consistency in these reports. There were no reports of increased breast cancer rates during periods of fat deprivation.

The National Institutes of Health (NIH) has finally launched their over one-half-billion-dollar, fifteen-year, 160,000-woman study on the effects of a low-fat diet on cancer and other health issues. Why not concentrate on finding out what actually happened to the millions of women who were forced to shift to a very low-fat diet during World War II? This would cost only a pittance and would certainly give immediate and highly useful insights into the problem. For all we know, the study has already been done and is moldering in a European library! We have noted the dramatic decrease in breast cancer in these women during and following the war. The evidence from Europe and all available published reports confirm this impression. I would trust the European World War II experience, where the fat reduction was universal, involuntary, profound, and prolonged, more than a study performed under artificial conditions. Why not spend the more than half a billion dollars on far less expensive and more effective health education to *prevent* breast cancer?

The surviving victims of Nazi concentration camps and the Japanese prisoner of war and internment camps reported cessation of menstrual periods coincident with caloric and fat restriction. Anecdotal reports attest to an absence of breast cancer. There can be no doubt that diet has a profound effect on hormones, and that these hormones have an equally powerful effect on the development of breast cancer.

## The Surgeon General's Report

In 1988, the U.S. Surgeon General released a massive report on the relationship between diet and health. It was officially called *The Surgeon General's Report on Nutrition and Health.*[62] Although other such studies had been previously attempted, this one was by far the most ambitious and important in medical history. It took over two hundred experts more than two years and quite a few million dollars to assemble virtually all of the world's credible scientific data on this vital issue.

*The report concluded that 60 percent of all cancers in American women were mostly or partially attributable to diet!* This amazing conclusion was the consensus of cautious, mainstream scientists speaking deliberately in full academic view. When the effects of alcohol were added, the effect was even more serious: "Together, these conditions account for as much as 70 percent of annual deaths among Americans." Their percentage does not include the effects of tobacco! The report further concluded that "most cancers have external causes and therefore are likely preventable."

For breast cancer, the report summarized thirty-two major studies, twenty-five of which supported the dietary fat, obesity, and breast cancer link for women. No studies showed a protective effect for fat. The studies that did not uphold the dietary connection had flaws in their methodology. These included self-reporting, limited range of fat exposure, limited range of ages, study group too small, and study period too brief.

The surgeon general's report's authors concluded that total caloric intake increased the risk of breast cancer, but not as much as fat intake. Protein excess and low fiber in the diet also increased the rates of breast cancer—but again, not as much as increasing the fat levels.

The 727-page volume is a gold mine of information on the vital subject of nutrition and health. It brought the subject fully into the mainstream of scientific inquiry and I think will ultimately be regarded as important as the 1964 *Surgeon General's Report on Tobacco and Health*. Yet, a May, 1992, request for the book from the U.S. Government Printing Office was returned with a rubber stamped OUT OF PRINT.

## What Does All This Mean?

It can never be conclusively proven that diet causes breast cancer. Similarly, it cannot be conclusively proven that smoking cigarettes causes lung cancer. Matters of this complexity cannot be easily demonstrated; it is unscientific and naive to suppose that they can be.

In both breast cancer and lung cancer, the totality of the evidence—the strength of the associations, the results of the animal studies, the effects of changing cultures and lifestyles, the consistency of the epidemiological studies, and the biological plausibility—combine to make the conclusion inescapable. The data is clear, consistent, and compelling. *Breast cancer is essentially a dietary disease*, just as lung cancer is essentially a smoking-related disease. Of course, there are exceptions to both statements, but they remain essential truths. There is more than sufficient evidence to warrant the appropriate changes now.

Many women feel that they can do nothing to prevent breast cancer. They are dangerously wrong. Breast cancer risk can be greatly reduced, and in individual cases eliminated, by dietary and lifestyle changes alone. The dietary change required is simple: *a switch from the traditional high-fat/low-fiber American diet to a low-fat/high-fiber diet.*

The seven countries with the highest rates of breast cancer (over 20 breast cancer deaths per 100,000 deaths in a year) are the very same countries where people eat the highest amounts of fat—150 grams (about a third of a pound) a day. By contrast, women who live in the seven countries with the lowest rates of breast cancer (less than 5 breast cancer deaths per 100,000 per year), eat the lowest amounts of dietary fat—less than 50 grams a day. Can this be a coincidence? I don't think so.

To understand fully the impact of dietary fat on the development of breast cancer, however, it is first necessary to learn how a high-fat diet affects hormone levels.

# 6

## The Estrogen Connection

*T*here is no doubt that estrogen plays a key role in the development of breast cancer. No matter how you analyze or approach the problem, hormones—chiefly estrogen—are the key components in the breast cancer riddle.

*Estrogen* is the dominant female hormone. *Progesterone* is the other, but it plays a lesser role in the development of breast cancer. The timing, strength, and duration of exposure to these hormones, combined with a genetic susceptibility, chiefly determine whether a woman will eventually develop cancer of the breast.

One of the obvious and overlooked proofs for the importance of estrogen is the rarity of breast cancer in males. There are at least one hundred female victims of breast cancer for every male. This is due to the lack of estrogen in males. It is often wrongly stated that the reason for the low incidence of breast cancer in males is their lack of breast tissue. The real reason is the lack of ovaries and therefore the lack of estrogen. It is also of interest that even among the male victims of breast cancer, the same risk factors apply as with females—primarily, a diet rich in fat. The highest recorded rate of male breast cancer is in western Germany, where the percentage of dietary calories from fat is a remarkably high 49 percent.

Among women who have surgically lost their ovaries, the risk of breast cancer is dramatically reduced. The earlier the loss, the less the probability of developing breast cancer. Such women are exposed to vastly less estrogen than women with normal ovaries even when provided with oral hormone replacement.

And among those women who eventually develop breast cancer, higher levels of active estrogen (the biologically active portion that is not bound to protein) are present, along with lower levels of an interfering substance called *sex-hormone-binding globulin* that works against estrogen.[63]

Estrogen apparently works as a breast cancer promoter on the cellular level. The details are not entirely understood, but it seems likely that the stimulation of the breast cells by estrogen results in an increase of abnormal cells that can become precursors to cancer. We do know that the majority of breast cancers arise in the cells of the terminal duct lobular unit. This is the portion of the breast where the glands and the ducts merge. Cells in this portion of the breast undergo dramatic changes during the two distinct phases of each menstrual cycle. The first part of this phase is dominated by estrogen acting mainly on the breast ducts, and the second by progesterone acting mainly on the glandular breast tissue. Natural progesterone, the progesterone produced by the ovary, protects against breast cancer. It is the *synthetic progestins* that have been linked with an increased incidence of breast cancer. The administration of natural progesterone (derived from Mexican yams) is an overlooked and protective therapy. It can reduce breast tenderness and "fibrocystic" changes as well as increase bone strength and thus protect against osteoporosis.

This gives rise to a concept of risk associated with the total number of menstrual cycles. It explains why both an early menarche (onset of menstruation) and a late menopause are risk factors for breast cancer. It also explains why women who lose ovarian function from disease or surgery have a reduced risk of breast cancer. A study from the National Cancer Institute demonstrated that a drop in total fat calories from 40 percent to 20 percent increased the length of the menstrual cycle by two days in two thirds of the subjects, thereby reducing the total number of cycles. Fewer cycles—for whatever reason—over a lifetime will result in a reduction of breast cancer risk.

As frequent as it may often seem to be, the menstrual cycle represents an important biological event—a woman's monthly preparation for pregnancy. An egg is released from the ovary, the lining of the uterus is prepared for the implantation and nourishment of the fertilized egg, and an intricate and delicate hormonal ballet follows. Among these changes are preparations *by the breast* for a pregnancy and for subsequent breast feeding. This is the reason for the premenstrual tenderness, swelling, and pain that most American women experience. It also seems to be related, at least in a general sense, to the subsequent development of breast cancer.

We have long known that although the risk of breast cancer is cumulative, the incidence rises less rapidly following menopause. Despite this, two thirds of all cases are in women over fifty years of age. Even though a woman's body produces lower levels of female hormones following menopause, she is still at increased risk if she is obese. Therefore, following menopause, obesity becomes a major risk factor.

Dietary fat and obesity tend to be markers for estrogen levels. Obese women are not only more likely to have higher levels of estrogen but also to have more menstrual disturbances. But while obesity is a strong risk factor after menopause, it seems to be a weak one before menopause. One possible explanation is that many young, obese women ovulate less frequently than women of normal weight and therefore have more episodes of lowered estrogen and progesterone levels. Obesity after menopause results in the production of large amounts of estrogen in the subcutaneous fatty tissues from a precursor material (called androstenedione) made in the adrenal glands (small glands located above each kidney). This source of estrogen is unrelated to ovarian production. Therefore, it is not unusual for young breast cancer patients to be slender when genetics are dominant in the causation of their disease, and it is common for postmenopausal women with breast cancer to be heavier than the average.

How does diet relate to estrogen and other hormones that are involved in the development of cancer? David Heber and his associates at the University of California, Los Angeles, School of Medicine placed women on a very low-fat diet (less than 10 percent of total calories) for only three weeks. In that short time the women experienced a profound drop— of 50 percent—in serum estradiol (a form of estrogen) levels. One patient dropped 80 percent.[64] A study from Boston measured hormone levels in the blood as well as the excretion of estrogen in vegetarian and meat-eating women. The results demonstrated dramatic differences in the patterns of estrogen metabolism. The vegetarian women had increased fecal excretion of estrogen, decreased levels of estrogen in the bile, and lower levels in the blood. The latter levels were 11 to 20 percent lower than those measured in the meat-eating women.[65] There are a large number of such essentially similar studies. Diet seems to be the main, controllable factor that moderates female hormone levels in the body and diet is therefore *the primary, controllable means of preventing breast cancer.*

*Prolactin* is another female hormone that is less well understood and studied than estrogen. As its name suggests, it is important in lactation. Its possible role in breast cancer is not fully known. However, there are prolactin receptors—sites on the surface of the cells that bind the hormone—in up to 40 percent of breast cancer cells, and several studies have shown a worsened prognosis in patients with high blood prolactin levels. Prolactin levels also respond to dietary measures. A study of women on a Western diet compared with those on a vegetarian diet[66] revealed decreased prolactin levels among the vegetarians. A similar study comparing Bantu women with white South African women revealed higher prolactin levels among the white women ingesting 40 percent of calories as fat compared with levels observed in the Bantus following a 15 percent fat diet.[67] In humans there seems to be a nighttime surge of prolactin. This prolactin surge is reduced by almost one-half on a vegetarian diet.[68] Elevated prolactin levels are associated with breast cancer in animals as well.

Dietary fiber also is related to estrogen levels in the blood. The higher the fiber content of the diet, the lower the estrogens in the blood. The fiber alters the extent of intestinal reabsorption of estrogen compounds and also helps the body eliminate estrogen compounds through the intestines. One of the first studies specifically to relate fiber to breast cancer was a 1986 article titled "Hypothesis: A New Look at Dietary Fiber." This study, noting that breast cancer was an estrogen-dependent disease, demonstrated that dietary fiber aids in the elimination of excess estrogen.[69]

A study of premenopausal women with cystic breast disease divided the women into two groups. One group was placed on a high-fiber diet using foods containing wheat, oat, and corn bran (thirty grams per day) while their fat levels were maintained at 36 percent of calories. They had significant drops in their estrone levels (estrone is one of three major estrogens in women). The other group's levels remained unchanged.[70]

The age of menarche is an important and interesting key

to the hormone riddle. The average age for menarche in the United States is currently 12.2 years. A hundred years ago, it was seventeen. In China today, the age is from fifteen to seventeen years. What is responsible for this dramatic difference? A clue can be found among the daughters and granddaughters of Chinese and other Asian women who are raised in America. They have the same early menarche as other young American women. Once again, this suggests that the difference is environmental and not genetic. It is also instructive to study the age of menarche in Japan. In 1875, that average age was 16.5. It gradually diminished to 13.9 years in 1950, and at present it is 12.6 years—about the same as in the United States. This is a classic example of a time-trend study. The only biologically plausible explanation for this dramatic shift is the substantial increase of dietary fat in Japan. Studies by T. Hirayama of the National Cancer Center Research Institute in Japan reveal a 4.2 times greater incidence of breast cancer in girls with onset of menses under thirteen years of age compared with those over seventeen years of age. Another clue to the source of early menarche is the greater body weight of girls with early puberty.[71] This weight increase is associated with a greater intake of fat, chiefly animal fat, during the developing years. Tallness is also related to such fat intake and has long been associated with an increased risk of breast cancer. "Why should being tall predispose a woman to breast cancer?" Chronically elevated hormone levels predispose to breast cancer, and just incidentally, to tallness as well.

The cattle industry's newsletter, the *Beef Brief,* reports that the Japanese are catching up to Americans in height: "The increases are attributed to greater consumption of beef burgers and other meats," according to a newsletter article entitled "Beefing Up in Japan. Eat Burgers, Grow Tall."[72] A review of the article in the *San Francisco Examiner* prompts the question: Will other Western ills follow? *They already*

**Age at First Menses as Related to Age Adjusted Breast Cancer Death Rates**

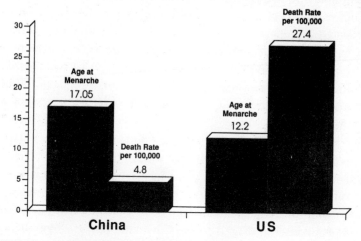

1. WHO Stastistics Annual quoted in *Clincal Oncology* American Cancer Society 1991, Atlanta, Georgia pg. 6.
2. *Breast Cancer: The Facts* Michael Baum 2nd edition 1988 Oxford University Press pg. 8.
3. T. Colin Campbell, *A Study On Diet Nutrition and Disease In The Peoples Republic of China*, 1990, Cornell University, Ithaca, New York pg. 5.

*have.* Heart attacks and prostate cancer, as well as a host of other diseases, have increased dramatically in Japan. The *Beef Brief* of October 1993 warns the public about the health risks of vegetarian diets and urges us to eat meat because it is good for the economy and good for the environment. Buyer beware when evaluating health advice from food-industry-sponsored publications.

To illustrate just how far this trend can develop, researchers at Duke University say that about half of the girls in America begin breast development and/or development of pubic hair *by age nine*. About 10 percent exhibit physical signs of puberty *by age seven*! Researcher Marcia Herman-Giddens analyzed 4,993 girls aged three to twelve years and hopes to study 20,000 such girls by the end of 1993.[73] Possible reasons given for the early puberty by the researchers included "better nutrition," "environmental causes," and "a number of factors we do not understand well at all." To attribute this disaster to better nutrition shows the hopelessness of much American thinking on the subject of nutrition. The real reason is that these unfortunate girls are provided a diet that is greatly overburdened with fat and protein. We have been conditioned to think of our nutrition as the safest and best in the world, when in truth it is among the most dangerous.

Contrast the findings of the Gidden study among Afro-American girls with the time of menarche in a native African tribe. The Kung girls of Africa menstruate for the first time, on average, at age 16.5 years.[74] This is also about the average time of marriage. They usually have their first child at about age nineteen and tend to bear five children, the last during the mother's mid-thirties. The birth of the last child is usually followed by menopause. Note the late menarche, the early menopause, and the very small number of menstrual cycles. It is no wonder that the Kung's breast cancer rates are among the lowest in the world.

The age of menarche is even later—17.1 years—in the Agta tribe in the Philippines. In Daly City, California, where 28 percent of the population is Filipino, I am told by my pediatric colleagues that the average age of menstruation among young Filipinas is not different from that of all other young girls in the city—about twelve years. By now the pattern should be abundantly clear: if young women are given natural diets, they experience menarche at around fifteen to seventeen years of age. With a high-fat Western diet, this age drops to between eleven and thirteen years.

What are we doing to our children? It is clear that we are literally bombarding their bodies with unrelenting, precocious, and dangerous hormone levels, which manifest themselves by this untimely, but easily measured, biological marker—menarche. It is this same, unrelenting hormonal pressure—caused by the standard American diet—working throughout the remainder of the woman's life that exposes her to an increased risk of breast cancer.

Our obsession with high-fat and fast-food diets is not only killing us, it is destroying the fabric of our society by allowing a crushing burden of illegitimacy to be possible. At the turn of the century in America, a young woman commencing her reproductive life at sixteen years and having her first child at, say, nineteen to twenty-one years, following her marriage, could become a responsible member of her societal group. A present-day girl, menstruating at eleven—*solely because of her diet*—and becoming pregnant and an unmarried mother at twelve or thirteen, represents two children in a great deal of trouble. And for that matter, a society in a great deal of trouble, with over two thirds of the live births in many cities being to such children. The reality is that children are having children, and the root cause is the diet of these children. There is no other valid explanation. It is not entirely due to their sexuality, although that is the commonly held belief. The young women studied by Dr. Shostak had the same patterns of sexual behavior, but they simply were unable to conceive due to their lack of sexual maturity.

Rapid growth during childhood has also been associated with a shortened life span. Mentioned earlier in Ross's experiments with rats, this phenomenon has been described in humans as long ago as 1959 in a *Journal of the American Medical Association* article by P. L. Krohn entitled "Rapid Growth, Short Life."[75] Other research supports this connection. The long-term trend in increasing height and weight parallels the decreasing age at menarche.[76] The measurement of height and weight is not as open to challenge as the age of menarche. Both seem due to nutritional factors.

At the other end of the reproductive span, the age at menopause is higher among U.S. women than it is among women living in countries with low breast cancer rates. The greater the total number of menstrual cycles experienced by a woman, it seems, the greater her risk of breast cancer. Clearly, the resulting increase in total duration of exposure to estrogen is a key factor in our high breast cancer rates.

Thus far, we have talked about the body's endogenous, natural, or internal hormone production. The other type of hormone exposure is exogenous, artificial, or external. Oral contraception represents a type of artificial hormone exposure. It is difficult to generalize about oral contraceptive agents because the formulations were substantially changed in the mid-1970s. The earlier oral contraceptives were sequential— during the first part of the menstrual cycle, estrogen was administered without an accompanying progesterone. A shorter second phase followed in which both estrogen and progesterone were taken. The final phase was withdrawal of all hormones. This type of administration led to increased levels of endometrial cancer (cancer of the inner lining of the uterus). This finding led to the development of the *unopposed estrogen* theory (increased risk of breast cancer from unrelenting estrogen administration). Modern oral contraceptives combine estrogen and progesterone. This virtually eliminates the unopposed estrogen effect and also has not only reduced endometrial cancer but actually seems to protect against it.

The newer combination-type oral contraceptives also seem to protect against ovarian cancer. These medications suppress ovulation and that seems to be the major reason for that protection. In addition, pregnancy also protects against ovarian cancer, possibly by reducing the total number of ovulations. This observation implies that something in the process of ovulating, or the body's "repair" of the ovarian surface following ovulation, predisposes a woman to the development of ovarian cancer.

However, the newer oral contraceptives do not show the same protection against breast cancer. On the contrary, contraceptive use leads to a small increase of risk of breast cancer for women under forty-five. The challenge for the pharmaceutical industry is to produce an oral contraceptive agent that is protective against *all* the hormonally sensitive tissues of the female body: the breasts, the ovaries, and the uterus.

## Hormone Replacement Therapy

The medical community has made an assumption that an increased risk of breast and uterine cancer is the price we must pay for preventing osteoporosis and heart disease through the administration of hormones. Postmenopausal hormone replacement therapy is by far the most important hormonal manipulation employed by American women. To maintain our global perspective, it is important to remember that very few women in the rest of the world are placed on hormone therapy as "treatment" for the menopausal state. And for that matter, who decided that menopause was a disease that required a medicine? Is this more of the "a pill for every ill" thinking that characterizes our present-day approach to medical care?

The first human application of hormone therapy was in 1896 by George Thomas Beatson of Glasgow, who reported three cases of advanced breast cancer that responded favorably to removal of the ovaries.[77] Three British surgeons, Drs. Boyd, Thompson, and Lett, reported similar findings between 1900 and 1905. In 1916, Drs. Lathrop and Loeb demonstrated that the removal of ovaries from mice prevented breast cancer.[78] It was not until the 1930s that researchers began fully to understand the relationship of estrogen to pregnancy and reproductive tumors. This was followed by the chemical isolation of estrogen and progesterone. The first injection of estrogen took place in 1931 and by 1938 powerful estrogen compounds were developed and in clinical use, but required injection. It must be mentioned that these products were initiated in an era when no safety testing was required. The injections were inconvenient and expensive, but by 1938 Schering Corporation chemists were able to synthesize a powerful new compound that could be taken in pill form. Unfortunately, another potent synthetic estrogen, DES, was isolated in Great Britain. That medication was found much later, in 1971, to be responsible for a number of fatal vaginal cancers in the daughters of women who had used DES while pregnant. This was the first clear evidence that estrogen could cause cancer even if the cancer was discovered in the patient's daughter.

Graham A. Colditz, M.D., of Harvard Medical School has written, "Breast cancer is caused by estrogens, both those produced by the body during the reproductive years and those added through the use of oral contraceptives and replacement hormone therapy." And, "the evidence overwhelmingly shows that current use increases the risk of breast cancer. For women over sixty, the use of replacement estrogens doubles the risk of breast cancer."[79]

As early as 1947 there were warning signs of the dangers of estrogen replacement. An article in the December 1947 *American Journal of Obstetrics and Gynecology* described premalignant changes and bleeding in the uterine lining of postmenopausal women who were using the newly discovered estrogen therapy. It was not until the 1970s that the increase in cancer of the uterus for women using hormone replacement therapy was fully documented. In the San Francisco Bay area, the incidence increased by 50 percent between 1969 and 1973. This resulted in an appropriate and precipitous decline in hormone replacement therapy. But after the formulations were modified, the use of these medications was gradually resumed.

Hormone replacement therapy (HRT) is used not only to treat menopausal symptoms, but also to protect against bone loss and heart disease. Millions of women take hormone replacement medications regularly. The net impact of this practice on the health of American women is hotly debated. There are more than fifty epidemiological and clinical studies as well as several meta-analyses (so-called super analyses that combine many smaller studies and are alleged to reveal otherwise undetectable differences) that have considered the relation of estrogen treatment to breast cancer risk. After reviewing much of this mountain of data, it is fair to say that there is no consensus. One can find evidence in the scientific literature to support *any* position on this question. This type of therapy is unique and quite recent in our medical history, and is in essence a giant medical experiment.

On balance, however, it seems well established that *prolonged estrogen usage does increase breast cancer risk*. There is still no agreement on which women should, or should not, take estrogen because of that increased risk. As with contraceptive pills, a problem in evaluating these studies is the change in estrogen formulations over the years. The drug industry and physicians responded to the alarming increases in endometrial cancer by reducing the dosage of the most commonly used estrogen by half. However, women receiving even this lowered dosage had approximately twice the level of endometrial (uterine) cancer as a similar woman without oral estrogen would have.

The problem in assessing the safety of estrogen use is the necessity to follow such patients for many years to determine the true risk. According to the North American Menopause Society, only about 15 percent of all American women receive hormone replacement therapy, and the average duration of that treatment is only nine months. Yet, after prolonged use of estrogen, breast cancer rates trend upward. The relative risk is 1.3 after fifteen years. In women with a positive family history for breast cancer, the risk is 3.4 times the average for women without hormone usage.[80]

Without the addition of synthetic progesterone-like

agents to the hormone replacement therapy, the risk of endometrial cancer is substantially increased. As mentioned, this resulted in a large increase of endometrial cancer following the almost routine use of HRT in the 1960s and 1970s. The initial response by the treating physicians was to sharply reduce the total amount of HRT. Later, progestins (*synthetic progesterone-like drugs*) were added to the formulations and the amount of estrogen was decreased. This combination of efforts sharply lowered the endometrial cancer incidence and mortality by the late 1970s. It was hoped that such combination therapy would also protect against breast cancer. But, sadly, the newer formulation seems to be resulting in a further increase in breast cancer. One prospective study from Sweden supports this association and describes a markedly increased risk among women receiving this combination.[81] The authors noted a 10 percent increase in the relative risk of breast cancer in 23,244 women receiving estrogens for menopausal symptoms. In addition to this, the risk increased sharply with increasing length of treatment. If the treatment lasted more than nine years, the excess risk was 70 percent. However, one must be very careful when evaluating data in this area. Older studies used chiefly conjugated equine estrogens (the most popular estrogen used in this country is extracted from *pre*gnant *mar*e's ur*ine*, hence the name "Premarin"). The European and Scandinavian studies use estradiol (or 17-Beta estradiol usually prepared from plant sources).

Synthetic, plant-derived estrogen is 17-Beta estradiol, the same as the natural estrogen that human females produce. There are four synthetic estrogens currently in common use. Studies of newer formulations do not have the long-term follow-up of the older, now obsolete studies. Such factors make the unbiased evaluation of hormone replacement therapy difficult.

Women who have had a hysterectomy do not have to

concern themselves with progesterone. But there is continuing debate among gynecologists as to the ideal method of administering progesterone for women whose uterus has not been removed. Some dosage methods result in postmenopausal women once again resuming menstrual periods. It should also be noted that the synthetic progestins do not have the same bone-preserving properties as estrogen or natural progesterone. They prevent bone loss in some areas of the skeleton containing a type of bone called *cortical*, but not in the spine that contains a type of bone called *trabecular*.[82]

It has been reported that postmenopausal women receiving hormone replacement therapy have a reduced risk of heart attack and stroke.[83] Yet other studies claim the opposite.[84] The Harvard Nurses' Study reported a reduced relative risk for heart disease, without specific mention of stroke.[85] The exact mechanism for such protection is not understood. There are favorable effects on total cholesterol, HDL, and LDL. Despite the confusion, most experts support the proposition that estrogen confers heart-protective benefits on American women. My recommendation after evaluating this bewildering array of data is to use hormone replacement therapy for relief of troublesome postmenopausal symptoms, but only for a reasonable period of time. Reasonable seems to be from five to seven years, although one could argue otherwise. I would counsel those who are not greatly troubled by postmenopausal symptoms (the chief symptom is flushing or "hot flashes"), and who wish to protect themselves from the problems of osteoporosis and heart disease, to seek this protection through improved nutrition (a low-fat, low-protein, high-fiber diet) and not through pills, tablets, or skin patches. It is unlikely that good health will come from a medicine bottle. If that were the case, how would we explain the striking lack of heart disease, osteoporosis, and cancer in areas of the world where these medications are not available? This observation deserves some additional comment. If you were to map out the parts of the world where women suffer most from osteoporosis, you would color in the United States, Canada, the United Kingdom, and Europe. These are the very parts of the world where the most estrogens, progestins, calcium pills, and milk are used. The parts of the world without a serious osteoporosis problem are the very countries where there is virtually no estrogen, progestins, calcium pills, or milk. Those countries include China, rural South America, and Africa. This irrefutable observation *must* be satisfactorily explained by advocates of dairy products, as well as estrogen and calcium supplementation.

Japanese menopausal women have infrequent and weak hot flashes compared with Western women. Although some have attributed this to "cultural indifference to the hot flush in Japan"[86], others decided to make more scientific measurements in Japan. A group of Finnish researchers compared the urinary concentrations of estrogen and phytoestrogens among Japanese, American, and Finnish women.[87] If a woman is efficiently eliminating excess estrogen, it appears in the urine. The Japanese women excreted one hundred to one thousand times more estrogen than American or Finnish women consuming a Western diet! (The likely cause for this pattern is the use of soy products including tofu, soybeans, and boiled beans.) These foods are weak estrogens (or phytoestrogens) and are thought to have biological effects during the menopause when estrogen levels are falling. This remarkable excretion of phytoestrogens may explain why hot flashes and other menopausal symptoms are so mild in Japanese women. It also helps to explain the powerful effect of diet on hormone-related diseases.

Among Americans, it has been observed that vegetarian women tend to have an earlier menopause than women who consume meat. Since early onset of periods and late menopause are risk factors for breast cancer, the vegetarian diet is seen as protective. Another factor already noted to protect against breast cancer is the increased level of dietary-fiber intake observed among vegetarian women. They usually ingest two or even two and a half times as much fiber as other American women eating a regular diet.

The evidence we've seen thus far tells us that breast cancer (as well as heart disease and osteoporosis) is chiefly a lifestyle-caused disease that is linked to hormone exposure, and that breast cancer can be prevented by changes in our dietary habits.

# Facts About Fats

*H*ow do fats affect hormone production, and hence, the development of breast cancer? Understanding some basic facts about fats will help clarify the issue.

Throughout this book we have almost always spoken of fat in a negative manner. There are a bewildering array of different fats, though, and there are different ways humans eat fat. What relationship do eating patterns have on health and longevity? How is breast cancer induced in animals? What is the ideal level of fat intake for humans? Is it the same at all ages? Are there good fats and bad fats? What are the recommendations of our health agencies?

First, we must recognize that the range of fat intake among the people of the world is enormous. At the lowest levels, we have records showing that the fat intake of Japanese soldiers in World War II accounted for as little as 3 percent of their total calories. At the other extreme, the entire population of western Germany is currently estimated to consume 49 percent of their total calories as fat. However, the most important numbers for you to keep in mind are the averages for total fat intake among American adults. This ranges from *34 to 44 percent of calories,* depending on which survey you read. American teenagers who eat many consecutive meals in fast-food restaurants can reach as much as 65 percent of their total calories as fat! We will be forced to face the full consequences of this behavior in the future. Individual meals that are extremely rich and unbalanced can total more than 80 percent of their calories as fat!

A commonsense and practical definition would describe fats as substances that are greasy to the touch, will not dissolve in water, but will dissolve in alcohol or ether. A chemical definition would include a listing of the structural components of fats. Fats are composed of only three basic elements: carbon, hydrogen, and oxygen. These happen to be the same elements that compose carbohydrates, but the amount of hydrogen is greater in the fats. Fat is found in all meat, oils, eggs, nuts, and dairy products except the nonfat variety.

Fats—or lipids—are the body's most concentrated sources of energy. Weight for weight, fat has more than twice the fuel value of either carbohydrates or protein (nine calories per gram, compared with four calories per gram for both protein and carbohydrates). Fats are readily stored by the human body, a fact that thirty-four million obese Americans deplore. It is difficult for the body to create fat deposits from protein and relatively difficult to make fat stores from carbohydrates.

Fats are not all bad. In fact, they are necessary for life itself. Without compounds containing fat, the development of the brain and nerve tissues during infancy would not be possible. The vital cell membranes depend on fats for their integrity, function, and as structural components. They are also part of the membranes that surround intracellular structures. The very structure of the sex hormones that we have spoken of in this book is based on fat molecules. Fat is also essential for the absorption of the fat-soluble vitamins: A, D, E, and K. Fat is also used by the body as insulation under our skin and for cushioning and shock absorption of our vital organs.

Why the fuss about fats if they're necessary for life? We Americans have gone to great excess in our intake of fat. As a result, we are becoming fatter and sicker. The human body simply cannot adapt to excessively high-fat diets, when chronically ingested. Even if you think that your diet is reasonable or balanced, if you are an average American in the 1990s, your fat intake is far in excess of safe limits. Remember that we established the average of total calories as fat in the American diet at 34 to 44 percent. All responsible experts agree that the American, or Western, diet with that level of fat intake is greatly elevated and extremely dangerous. To turn the matter around, it is virtually impossible to design an adult diet that is truly fat *deficient*. The amount of essential fat required is almost vanishingly small, less than 2 percent of calories. Only a diet based entirely on fruit would be likely to result in fat deficiencies.

*Cholesterol* is the type of fat most often mentioned when heart and vascular disease is considered. However, it is not a major factor in breast cancer causation and we will not dwell on it, or its components, HDL, LDL, or triglycerides. Do not be misled by marketing strategies that proclaim that a food is noncholesterol when it is a nonanimal fat. *All* vegetable oils are noncholesterol even though they are 100-percent fat. This dishonest marketing tactic has been duping American shoppers for years. *Cholesterol comes only from animal sources*. Noncholesterol products can still be 100 percent fat and very damaging to your health. Besides, much of the cholesterol in our body is produced by our own bodies in response to noncholesterol fats.

Scientists group the fats into three categories: saturated fat, monounsaturated fat, and polyunsaturated fat. It may be helpful to define the term *saturated*. If you can visualize fat molecules as chains of carbon atoms that are linked together with bonds, it will become understandable. Carbon is an element, one of 109 such substances that are indivisible except by nuclear reactions. But carbon is the only element that can join together in short or long chains or rings that function as backbones of a larger unit, the molecule. Each carbon atom has four bonding sites, like little hooks or magnets. Usually, they are used to bond to other carbon atoms, hydrogen atoms, elements, or other chemical compounds. Because of this unique ability, the number of carbon compounds is larger than the number of compounds involving all other elements. If there is an unused bonding site, it usually lines up between two carbon atoms on the long carbon chain. This becomes a point of possible attachment of another atom or group of atoms that will cause saturation.

If there are no unused (or "double") bonds, the fat is said to be *saturated*. If there is only *one* such bond, it is *monounsaturated*. If there are many such bonds, the fat is considered *polyunsaturated*. It's as simple as that (there can be from one to six double bonds in a carbon chain). Why should we bother talking about double bonds? It seems that they determine the biological functions and properties of the fatty acids.

*Saturated* fats are those that are predominantly solid or hard at room temperatures. These fats chiefly originate from animal sources such as lard, beef, pork, lamb, butter, whole milk, and cream. Only two vegetable fats have high percentages of saturated fat: palm and coconut oils. One way that vegetable fats can become solid is through the process of *hydrogenation*. This is a chemical process that converts liquid vegetable oils into solids or semisolids. Avoid hydrogenated products whenever you can. In general, the saturated fats are thought to be causative agents for heart disease, and to a lesser extent, for cancer.

*Monounsaturated* fats are chiefly found as olive oil and one of the fats present in beef.

*Polyunsaturated* fats are liquid oils that come from vegetables, oils, and seeds. They include: corn, safflower, soybean, peanut, cottonseed, rapeseed, sunflower, and sesame-seed oils. We noted earlier the remarkable increase in consumption of these oils in America since the mid-1960s.

Fats are usually mixtures of the various types with one type predominating. For example, safflower oil contains 8-percent saturated, 13-percent monounsaturated, and 79-percent polyunsaturated fat. Safflower oil is thus most accurately classified as a polyunsaturated fat.

Fats are occasionally referred to as omega-3 fats, omega-6 fats, or omega-9 fats. Omega is the last letter of the Greek alphabet, and the omega number is based on the location of the first double bond when counting carbon atoms from the methyl, or left, end of the fat molecule. The fats differ in their biochemical behavior depending on the location of that bond. So don't be intimidated when you hear of an omega-6 fat. In general, the omega-3 fats are the more beneficial of the fats, and the omega-6 less so, and the omega-9 fats least of all. The saturated fats have no double bonds and therefore no omega numbers.

Some fats are referred to as *essential*. This means that the human body cannot manufacture that fat, and its absence will create a deficiency. Essential fats can only come from an outside food source. Linoleic acid and linolenic acid are the most common essential fats and are found in certain vegetable, seed, and nut oils. Essential fats are primarily derived from plant-based foods. They are synthesized in a part of plants (the chloroplasts) and probably also by algae. Only plants possess the enzymes to insert double bonds into fatty acids at the specific spots necessary to create essential fatty acids. The richest available pure source of linoleic acid is flaxseed oil.

If fat is involved in the genesis of breast cancer, we have to decide which of the above fats are the most dangerous, and whether or not there are any "good" fats. Though animal or saturated fats are most implicated in the initiation of coronary artery disease and stroke, vegetable sources of polyunsaturated fat, often thought to be free of harmful effects, can be involved with cancer formation. I realize that this is a very unsettling notion to most people, who have been told for years that the lovely, clear, yellow oils that are sold in glass or plastic containers are health foods. The evidence, however, supports the probability that they are contributors to breast cancer and prostate cancer as well as to other malignancies. Olive oil has the least enhancing effect on breast cancer growth, and there is some evidence that fish oils may actually be protective.[88, 89]

Our prehistoric ancestors did not have access to concentrated vegetable oils. The *Encyclopedia Britannica*[90] puts the earliest use of vegetable oils at 2500 B.C. The practice of frying food submerged in hot oil was first described in an English reference of 1290 A.D.[91] In this country, the widespread and heavy usage of vegetable oils came only after the dangers of cholesterol and saturated fats were recognized in the 1950s and 1960s. In an effort to keep the American diet as unchanged and as rich as possible, vegetable oils were described as the good fats, and their use soared. Steady increases in breast, colon, pancreatic, and prostatic cancer followed after several years. In my opinion, these increases are substantially related to the increase in consumption of oils and hydrogenated fats. Yet we must not lose sight of the fact that it is the *total* fat intake that best correlates with cancer levels in nearly every country studied.

In animal experiments, there is no doubt that vegetable oils are the most potent breast cancer promoters. Polyunsaturated vegetable oils promote cancer more effectively than either saturated fats or fish oils. It has been known for over seventy-five years that mice or rats fed such diets spontaneously develop breast cancer far more readily and often than animals fed low-fat diets. Most texts cite the work of A. Tannenbaum in the 1940s as the first to make this association. I found that Kanematsu Sugiura at what later became the Sloan-Kettering Institute was doing work in this area as early as 1917.[92] The doctors of that time scoffed at the idea of "starving" an already weakened cancer patient. This was consistent with the long-held belief in American medicine that the linking of dietary habits with cancer was quackery. This relationship is less clear with humans; it seems that the *total* dietary fat content relates more closely to breast cancer incidence than any specific type of fat.[93]

Scientists who performed animal experiments found a method to rapidly induce breast cancer, chiefly in mice and rats. Such animals with breast cancer could then be exposed to dietary manipulations or various treatments in an effort to gain insights that would be helpful in combating human breast cancer. The method is worth mentioning briefly, as it may have some parallels in human breast cancer induction. The animals are fed a dose of a chemical called DMBA. DMBA is an abbreviation of dimethylbenzanthracene, which is a fat-soluble hydrocarbon compound. Because of its solubility in fat, it accumulates and persists in the fatty tissue of the mammary glands and thereby greatly increases the exposure of the animal's breast tissue to the cancer-causing DMBA. Another chemical, N-nitrosomethylurea, or NMU, has similar action in causing breast cancer to develop promptly in mice and rats. Researchers who believe that pesticides are involved in the genesis of human breast cancer feel that the pesticides accumulate and act in a manner quite similar to that described for DMBA and NMU above. The full story of the pesticide issue has not yet been told, but I can give you some reasonable advice in the meanwhile. *Stay away from pesticides whenever possible.* This means carefully washing foods, avoiding direct contact with pesticides, but far more importantly, avoiding animal fats and dairy fat where the pesticides concentrate. Pesticides are "lipophilic," which means that they concentrate in fatty foods. To avoid them, eat low on the food chain; keep to a plant-based diet.

Based on a review of the scientific literature on the subject of fat and cancer, I have concluded that the use of oxidized, hydrogenated, and processed fats is a major factor causing breast cancer for American women. If this thinking is correct, a logical question would be: "How do these fats damage cells and cause cancer?" It is well established that polyunsaturated fats and hydrogenated fats have a deleterious effect on the membranes of our cells. Cell walls or cell membranes (also called plasma membranes) are transparent and microscopically thin (0.005 micrometers). They enclose every living cell. This is probably the most important surface, or interface, in all of biology. Fats and fatty acids have an important part in the normal functioning as well as the structure of the cell membrane. In fact, they actually become incorporated into the cell membrane. The fat in the cell walls regulates the delicate electrical charges that allow the orderly movement of minerals, oxygen, and hormones into and out of the cells. *If these fats have been altered by processing and hydrogenation, they still become incorporated into the cell wall, but then the cell will function abnormally.*[94]

It is across this microscopically thin barrier that large, water-soluble molecules and electrically charged particles called ions must be transported to the interior of the cell. Proteins within the lining membrane act as pumps and force needed nutrients into the interior of the cell. A well-functioning cell membrane can pump elements such as potassium into the cell and elements such as sodium out of the cell. Other particles too large to be pumped are either swallowed into or disgorged from the cell by an opening and closing off of the membrane. The vital cell membrane, when functioning normally, can correct abnormalities in the amount of these substances by transporting particles out of and into the cell.

The fats mentioned above and *free radicals* (chemically unstable substances) damage the cell membrane and cause it to become both leaky and stiff. This results in a general dysfunction of the cell. This invisible cell membrane layer is absolutely critical to life and health. With trillions of cells in our bodies, it is unwise to ingest any substance that could damage these delicate and essential cell membranes.

This cellular dysfunction may partially explain the effect of fat on immune function. We have long known that a high-fat diet partially "paralyzes" or suppresses the immune system. Vegetable fats are also immunosuppressive and, by the effect of inhibition, can contribute to the development of cancer. Lymphocytes or white blood cells are highly active in living cell cultures. In special phased-light microscopic preparations, they can actually be seen destroying abnormal or invading cells, bacteria, and even cancerous cells. It seems certain that at least part of the deleterious effect of fat on these protective white blood cells is to damage their cellular membranes and render them less effective. Many respected cancer researchers believe that every person produces cancerous cells in the normal process of repair and growth. Normally functioning lymphocytes destroy or isolate those cells. It is a reasonable hypothesis that the increase of breast cancer is not only due to cancer-causing substances, but also to the inability of damaged lymphocytes to destroy cancer cells. Recent research suggests that low-fat diets boost overall cancer immunity. On the other hand, people following diets that are high in fats and oils have less ability to suppress cancer cells. The "natural killer" cell count is depressed in such people.[95] A commonplace observation among patients who switch to a very low-fat diet is: "I just don't get colds anymore."

In addition to damage from polyunsaturated fats and hydrogenated fats, our bodies' delicate cell membranes are also damaged by free radicals, those troublesome substances we mentioned earlier that can also attack, stiffen, and harm the cell membranes much as the hydrogenated compounds can. Free radicals are chemical substances that have an unpaired or odd number of electrons in their atomic makeup. This creates a chemical instability and creates a higher energy level as the atom attempts to either give up, or acquire, an electron in order to achieve stability. If we think of an atom as a miniature solar system, the nucleus, or center, of the atom would be like the sun and the electrons would be similar to orbiting planets. If an energy source impacts the atom, an electron can be forced out of orbit. This makes that atom unstable and capable of delivering a high energy. This molecule becomes a free radical. It will eagerly transfer that electron, with its damaging energy, to any nearby substance that will receive it. Electrons are more stable when paired. Free radicals are therefore considered highly reactive and volatile.[96] Although free radicals are present in normal biochemical reactions, their numbers must be kept under control. They tend to be increased by the normal process of oxidation, or burning of fuel in the body, for energy. In addition to that, exposure to various toxins such as cigarette smoke, industrial solvents, excessive sunlight, or smoked foods generate additional free radicals. Damage to cells results.

Through a complex series of steps, polyunsaturated fats promote the production of free radicals and become incorporated into cell membranes, which then are more easily damaged.[97] Polyunsaturated fats also contribute to another harmful process to be explained below—oxidation. It is believed that these events, over a span of years, can lead to the development of cancer. Free radicals can also damage the nucleus of the cell and thus damage the DNA and genetic material contained within it. This damage can lead to alterations of the genetic programming of that cell and predispose it to subsequent cancer formation. Danish scientists have been able to measure an indicator of DNA oxidation in the urine of cigarette smokers. It is felt that the formation of the free radicals is linked to the known increase in smokers' metabolic rates.[98] Oxidation is also important to an understanding of the role of fats and oils in disease.[99] Unsaturated oils oxidize readily. In so doing, they produce large amounts of free radicals. Although oxygen is essential to life, the normal metabolism of oxygen can produce very toxic by-products including free radicals and *singlet* oxygen, which is not technically a free radical but acts as one. Earlier we referred to the natural *antioxidants* as vitamin C, vitamin E, and the beta-carotenes. (Vitamin C is water-soluble, while vitamin E and the beta-carotenes are fat-soluble.) Our bodies need both types of antioxidants to protect the watery portions of the body as well as the more oily cell membranes. Antioxidants counteract the harmful effects of free radicals, by absorbing, neutralizing, or competing for the free radicals and thereby reducing their dangerous effects.

Beta-carotene (*pro-vitamin* A) is the real vitamin A, and is probably the most efficient of the antioxidants. Unfortunately, it is eaten in only small amounts by most Americans. The United States Department of Agriculture Food Intake Survey shows that the average American eats only 1.5 milligrams a day of beta-carotene. Carrots are the most common but only one of the best sources of beta-carotene: others include sweet potatoes, squash, leafy greens, chard, kale, broccoli, spinach, pumpkin, peaches, persimmons, cantaloupe, papaya, mangoes, tomatoes, and apricots. All of these foods have a deep orange, yellow, red, or green pigmentation. Drinking fresh juice made from vegetables rich in beta-carotene will accomplish the same goal, as will supplements. Some of the beta-carotene taken in will be converted by your body to vitamin A, and the body seems to have its own wisdom in determining the correct amount of beta-carotene to be converted.

The Physician's Health Study is a ten-year study of over

22,000 male physicians. Those with a history of heart disease had a greatly reduced incidence of further heart problems, strokes, and cancers when they took fifty milligrams of beta-carotene on alternate days, compared with those who took a placebo (an inactive substance).[100] Another Harvard study with a much larger group of subjects, this time women, found a lowered risk of stroke and heart disease among those women with a higher beta-carotene intake. Current thinking concerning the protective effects of beta-carotene holds that the same biochemical actions that protect the cells against cancer also prevent damage to the arterial walls that can lead to strokes and heart attacks.

The next antioxidant, vitamin C, is found in citrus fruits and juices, melons, leafy greens, cruciferous vegetables, green and red peppers, papaya, mangoes, berries, and tomatoes. Note that many of these foods also contain beta-carotene. Vitamin C is water-soluble and the body will eliminate the portion not needed; thus excessive bodily levels are not a problem. However, the body cannot store vitamin C and it is necessary to consume it daily. A variety of studies have shown protective effects from vitamin C against the development of heart disease and certain cancers. In a review of twelve major studies concerning nutrition and breast cancer, Howe and his associates found that vitamin C had the most consistent protective effect in preventing breast cancer of the various dietary factors studied.[101]

Vitamin E completes the list of antioxidants. Just as with the beta-carotenes and vitamin C, the use of vitamin E appears to reduce the risk of heart disease and cancer.[102] Vitamin E is found in seeds, nuts, wheat germ, leafy greens, mangoes, and certain oils. Cells have both aqueous, or water-soluble, and lipid, or fat-soluble, compartments. Vitamin E operates in the fat-soluble or lipid compartment of cells. Here it can break the chain reaction of oxidation that damages the plasma membrane.[103, 104] You *can* overdose on vitamin E, or any other fat-soluble vitamin. A reasonable dosage for supplementation is four hundred to eight hundred I.U. per day.

We have known for years that persons who eat a diet rich in grains, legumes, vegetables, and fruits have a lowered risk of cancer. Some experts feel that the best approach is to combine the eating of these protective foods while supplementing them with the cancer-preventing compounds listed here.

There is one more confusing and relatively new area of research and concern in the area of fats. This is the subject of "*trans-*"fats or *trans*-fatty acids. *Trans*-fatty acids are formed during the process of hardening vegetable oil from liquids into spreads or solid sticks through *hydrogenation.* Liquid oils have not been hydrogenated and therefore contain no *trans*-fats. Human beings can synthesize only *cis*-fatty acids (the opposite of *trans*-fatty acids); only bacteria can synthesize *trans*-fatty acids. The *trans*-fats can be used as fuel but they accumulate in cell substances called phospholipids with partially known, but almost certainly bad, results. Fortunately, *trans*-fats are not an extremely large part of our fat intake, but even small amounts of harmful substances are a cause for concern. Common dietary sources of *trans*-fats are margarines, cookies, biscuits, cake, and white bread. The women in a Harvard study[105] took in less than 10 percent of their calories as *trans*-fats. Yet those of the 85,000 middle-aged women who ate more than four pats of margarine a day were 50 percent more likely to be victims of heart disease than those who avoided it altogether. In the United States, the main source of *trans*-fats is partial hydrogenation.[106] The food industry loves *trans*-fats because they are more stable and have a greater shelf life. But this will not translate into a longer life for the humans who eat those fats.

Are there any fats that we can recommend as cancer preventive agents? Probably not, except in very small amounts. There are two fats, though, that are the least dangerous. They are the monounsaturated fats (the type found in olive oil) and omega-3 fats and oils (found chiefly in fish).

We know that fish oils protect against development of breast cancer in animals. Little work has been done in relating this observation to humans. Kaizer and his associates compared international breast cancer incidence and mortality rates against consumption of fish as well as other foods and nutrients. They found a consistent protective effect, suggesting that the omega-3 fatty acids contained in fish may protect against breast cancer.[107] These omega-3 oils derive from plankton, the bottom rung of the marine food ladder that nourishes all fish. One theory holds that the omega-3 oils have "antifreeze" properties that allow these fish to live in the frigid waters of the North Pacific and Atlantic Oceans. Omega-3 oils are important in the functioning of another group of molecules called the prostaglandins. These substances have a great deal to do with the reduction of inflammation and the promotion of healing in the body as well as the reduction of spasm or increasing the relaxation of blood vessels. They are also involved in reducing excessive clotting, as well as combating tumor growth and allergic reactions.

Flaxseed oil is another beneficial type of oil with an extremely high ratio of the essential fat, linolenic acid. It should only be used cold, not for cooking, and in small amounts. Advocates of flaxseed oil supplementation recommend one, or at the most, two teaspoons per day. Our main source of linolenic acid should be green and leafy vegetables.

## Consuming Meat and Dairy Products

Any discussion of fat must deal directly with the question of eating meat. We teach our children from their earliest years to eat far too much meat. Even though beef consumption has dropped 13 percent since 1980, Americans still eat sixty-five pounds per person per year, and it remains our most popular meat. We have made up for our reduction in beef consumption by greatly increasing our intake of poultry and fish. Despite this, hamburger is still America's largest single source of fat. One survey reported that between the ages of seven and thirteen years, our children average over six hamburgers a week.

Since this dietary pattern starts in early life, it may explain why children ten years of age or younger who died in accidents were found at autopsy to have arterial degeneration. An even more alarming development is the finding that a few children in their early teens required surgery to unblock the clogged carotid arteries that supply blood to the brain. We first had this unpleasant reality brought to our attention during the Korean conflict when autopsy studies of fallen American soldiers were compared with the findings of autopsy results in Korean soldiers. The pathologists were horrified to find arteriosclerosis to be universal and severe among the Americans, but virtually absent in the Koreans. This tragic finding was reconfirmed during the Vietnam conflict.

It must be remembered, though, that very young children need some fat and some cholesterol until they reach two years of age. These substances are necessary for the proper development and maturation of the brain and nerve tissues. Yet it is of interest that infants raised on soy-based formulas do not develop clinical hypocholesterolemia (or low cholesterol). We should also recall that in 1950 the Japanese nation had a total fat consumption of only 7.5 percent of total calories. This strikingly low level certainly did not prevent the Japanese from developing normal intelligence and nervous system function.[108] As for the adults, according to Jeremy Rifkin in *Beyond Beef*[109], the average middle-class American consumes over a ton of grain each year, but four fifths of that grain is consumed indirectly by eating grain-fed animals. Asian adults consume only three hundred to four hundred pounds of grain per year, almost all of it directly. (The average Asian consumes only eight grams of animal protein per day, while the average American consumes sixty-six grams or more of animal protein out of a total of over one hundred grams.)

A typical American adult will eat the meat of seven 1,100 pound steers in his or her lifetime! This is based on 65 pounds of meat a year and 659 pounds of dressed meat per 1,105-pound steer. Another source says that annual consumption of red meat and poultry is much higher, at 178 pounds per person. Each year the average American family of four eats half a steer, a whole pig, 100 chickens, 556 eggs, and 280 gallons of milk products, according to this source. Over an entire lifetime, the average American eats the flesh of 15 cows, 211 hogs, 900 chickens, 12 sheep, multiple thousands of eggs, hundreds of gallons of milk and ice cream, hundreds of pounds of cheese and saturated fats in the form of butter, margarine, and lard.[110] Because of their high-fat content, meat and dairy products provide the most significant source of dietary fat in the American diet. As a result, their impact on the development of breast and other diet-related cancers cannot be ignored. Combined with our use of added fats and oils previously discussed, the American diet presents a recipe for breast cancer.

Interestingly enough, our awareness of the deleterious effects of a diet rich in fats dates back to biblical times. Do you remember the story of Daniel, who was forced into King Nebuchadnezzar's court? He resolved not to eat the "King's food," which was described as "meat and wine" in the Old Testament. He kept his health by maintaining his customary diet of peas, beans, lentils, and water ("pulses and water" in the King James Version). Read the first chapter of Daniel for an intriguing account of what probably was the first controlled experiment in human nutrition with an emphasis on meat. Old Testament scholars estimate the time of this story at about 165 to 160 B.C. The story leaves a bit of doubt as to whether Daniel became ill as a result of eating the king's food. Most students gain the impression that he did.

Throughout history, gout was the "disease of kings and queens," the only people rich enough to eat meat at every meal. The first author to write specifically on the matter of prevention of cancer by dietary means was an Englishman, William Lambe, in an 1809 book with the ponderous title *Report on the Effects of a Peculiar Regimen on Scirrhous Tumors and Cancerous Ulcers*. He clearly states that persons with high meat intakes had higher cancer rates. A *Scientific American* article in January, 1892 noted that cancer was "most frequent among those branches of the human race where carnivorous habits prevail."

Only a few years later, in 1907, a remarkable study was reported in *The New York Times*. This study contrasted the eating habits of various ethnic groups in Chicago. The Germans, Irish, and Scandinavians were described as heavy meat eaters and had high rates of death from cancer. The Italians and Chinese, by contrast, relied more on pasta or rice, had lower intakes of meat, and had lower rates of cancer. The survey was not sophisticated by contemporary standards, but it did include 4,600 cases in a seven-year period from 1900 to 1907, and must rank as one of our earliest efforts at putting numbers to what we all now know to be true.

In England, in 1916, Rolo Russell wrote a book entitled *Notes on the Causation of Cancer*. His thesis was that cancer mortality was highest "in countries that eat more flesh."

During this same period, it was noted that cancer rates fell in Europe during and after World War I. During that emergency, meat and fats were almost totally unavailable. In Denmark, the death rate from non–war-related disease fell by 34 percent.[111] It was nearly seventy years before modern and more sophisticated epidemiological studies fully confirmed these early impressions.

During the Second World War, the same situation was once more observed, but this time the record keeping was far better and the conclusions more secure. Many millions of European and English women were forced into following a diet containing very little meat and almost no added fat. Cancers and heart attacks were both greatly reduced and remained so until a full seven or eight years following the war. The importance of this observation cannot be overstressed. We know that these women followed low-fat diets. In modern studies, this cannot be verified, or the range of fat ingestion is too narrow and too high to give meaningful data. However, one study in Hawaii found that animal fat and protein, especially from sausage, processed cold cuts, beef, lamb, and whole-milk dairy products was associated with the highest rates of breast cancer.[112] The average American eats 70 or more grams of animal protein each day, out of a total protein intake of 107 grams or more. In Asia, the story is far different. Out of a total of only fifty-six grams of protein, a mere eight is from animal sources. The incidence of breast cancer varies directly with the total amount of animal protein eaten, until very high levels are reached and "saturation" takes place. Following this, additional amounts of protein and accompanying fat appear to make little difference.

Meat is also devoid of fiber and this contributes to elevated hormone levels by reducing the fecal excretion of estrogen. High protein levels in childhood cause rapid maturation, early menarche, greater body weight, increased tallness, and more breast cancer.[113] High protein levels are not associated with increased longevity. Although the world is in love with tallness, premature and abnormal tallness in young children, in the absence of genetic reasons, represents a danger. This condition is often associated with an excess of fats and total calories in the child's diet.

## Safety of Our Meat Supply

How is meat implicated in cancer formation? Certainly the high fat and cholesterol associated with animal proteins are well-known factors. Less well-known is the fact that hormones given to the animal during life can persist after the death of the animal and are consumed with the meat. It's profitable to use hormones to raise cattle: hormones make the animal heavier and "tender." Commercial estrogens will increase daily weight gain of animals by 8 to 15 percent and improve feed efficiency by 5 to 10 percent in beef cattle or lambs.[114] In 1988, the European Economic Community banned the use of anabolic substances such as testosterone, progesterone, and estradiol-17 in animal production. They also banned the importation of U.S. beef treated with these substances. In fairness, it must be said that some of the prohibition of meat sales where hormones are used is more economically and politically than medically motivated.

Pesticides, bacterial, and viral contamination are too often present in the meat that we consume. The pesticide issue, in particular, deserves serious consideration. One researcher, Frank Falck, found high levels of PCBs and DDEs in the fatty breast tissue of women with breast cancer compared with similar tissue in women with benign breast disease (DDE is the end product of DDT metabolism).[115] Falck believes that these chemicals become concentrated in human fatty tissue, as in the breast, and act as co-carcinogens or promoting agents, and thus may play a role in breast cancer risk. Other research suggests that a variety of chemicals, including pesticides, may have an estrogenlike effect in a woman's body. It is possible that the high levels of pesticide found in the women's breast tissue may have resulted from years of ingesting pesticide-laden animal fats.[116] The pesticide residue that accumulates in the fat of animals also becomes lodged in the fatty tissue in a woman's breast.[117]

Although many dedicated and sincere activists are certain that pesticides and chemicals are the sole cause of breast cancer, I do not believe this conclusion is fully warranted. In California, agricultural regions and counties with the greatest exposure to pesticides have the lowest rates of breast cancer.[118] The island state of Sri Lanka, formerly Ceylon, was sprayed with thousands of tons of DDT following World War II. Malaria was virtually eradicated. However, the breast cancer rates were low before the pesticide exposure and have remained low.[119] Animal experimentation does not require the addition of pesticides to fat in order to cause breast cancer. A change in diet alone, without consideration of pesticides and chemicals, is sufficient to greatly reduce hormone levels in humans. These observations and a negative large-scale study from the Kaiser Health Foundation at least cast some doubt on the uncritical acceptance of the pesticide/breast cancer link. Yet these are dangerous compounds and must be eliminated or greatly reduced. I believe that any effect of organochlorines or other pesticides and chemicals is made possible by the high-fat diet which carries at least 90 percent of these lipophilic—or fat-seeking—materials, into a woman's body.

Bacterial contamination of our meat supply is of equal concern. The E. coli O157:H7 bacterial contamination of fast-food hamburgers cost three children their lives in 1993.[120] In the early days of this century, *The Jungle* by Upton Sinclair shocked this country with its description of filthy conditions in slaughterhouses. Although the book stimulated some reform in 1906, unsanitary conditions have never been eliminated. Rifkin's *Beyond Beef* has reopened discussion of this problem. When people get sick from eating contaminated meat, the USDA tends to blame the victims, or the food preparers, for details of refrigeration or cooking. My concern would not only be the method of food preparation but the far more important issue of how the E. coli poisoned the meat in the first place. To put it bluntly, why did fecal material get into the meat? That is the important issue, not the details of the housewife's skillet temperature. Even toxoplasmosis, an almost forgotten disease, is making a comeback when contaminated meat is not heated sufficiently.[121]

There is also a very considerable incidence of bovine leukemia present in American cattle herds. When confronted with this problem, other countries—Switzerland and Germany, for example—addressed it directly and have long been culling their herds of the leukemic cattle. In this country, and in parts of South America, it appears that governments have chosen to conceal the problem. One survey showed that 60 percent of American dairy cows are now infected. This results in an even higher percentage of the pooled milk being contaminated by admixture. A disturbing 1992 Colorado State study not only showed 52 percent of a dairy cattle herd positive for the bovine leukemia virus, but it also demonstrated that 21 percent of the same herd were positive for the bovine AIDS virus, or the bovine immunodeficiency virus (BIV).[122] Of course, the milk is eventually pasteurized and presumably the virus is inactivated. However, I find it disturbing to consider drinking milk containing bovine leukemia and immunodeficiency viruses, even if those viruses have allegedly been killed.[123, 124]

Milk is the only common food so contaminated with bacteria and viruses that we must sterilize it (pasteurize it) before it can be safely ingested. This fact alone should make one uneasy about the American pattern of heavy milk intake. Some other foodstuffs that pose a bacterial hazard in addition to milk are hot dogs, ground meats, soft cheeses, undercooked chicken, and raw fish.

On November 5, 1993, a decade of bitter controversy was ended as the Food and Drug Administration approved a genetically engineered hormone called bovine growth hormone (BGH). This hormone, when injected into dairy cows, increases milk production by as much as 25 percent. Unfortunately, it also causes more infections in treated cows and therefore requires more administration of antibiotics to those animals, the residues of which are then consumed by the persons drinking the milk. The widespread use of this hormone is also questionable on economic grounds, as the American public is already paying farmers for an excess milk supply. The most unpleasant aspect of the growth hormone affair, is that the FDA will not require labeling of the milk from BGH-treated cows. In fact, the dairy companies may not voluntarily label their product BGH free!

There are other problems associated with beef. In England in 1985, a puzzling cow's disease called "mad cow" disease or bovine spongiform encephalopathy (BSE) was discovered. This dreadful disease attacks the brains of cows and is uniformly fatal. The current rate of infection in England is greater than 850 cows per week. Since 1985, more than 120,000 cows have been diagnosed with mad cow disease, then killed, and their bodies destroyed by incineration as required by British law![125] As a result of this, beef consumption has fallen by about 25 percent and more than two thousand British schools have stopped serving beef to their children.

Returning to a discussion of the bovine leukemia virus, the virus is not only found in the milk of affected cattle, but in the meat also (although it is presumably killed by cooking). While no proof currently exists that humans can contract cancer from meat viruses, it is more probable that there can be an eventual reduction of resistance to lymphomas (a type of lymphatic cancer) when beef and cows' milk is consistently eaten and drunk over many years.

## Meat Consumption and Cancer Development

In an article published in the *Lancet*—"Lymphomas and Animal-Protein Consumption"[126]—Dr. Allan S. Cunningham described milk as "liquid meat" and tracked both milk and meat consumption (in grams per day) in fifteen countries for a one-year period. New Zealand, the United States, and Canada were the highest in that ranking. The lowest was Japan, followed by Yugoslavia and France. The difference between the highest and lowest intakes of beef and milk was striking. For example, New Zealanders ingest nearly thirty times more beef and milk than the Japanese. *There was a highly significant positive correlation between deaths from lymphomas and beef/dairy ingestion in all fifteen countries analyzed.*

This type of information, although not proving causation, must not be ignored. Dr. Cunningham feels that there *is* a causal link. He believes that the chronic absorption of animal-protein fragments into the human circulation stimulates excessive antibody production, which, after many years, finally overwhelms the human immune system, resulting in lymphomas.

The association between milk use and lymphoma incidence was also noted in Norway[127] where two or more glasses of milk daily—or the equivalent in dairy products—created odds 3.4 times greater of developing lymphoma than those in persons drinking less than one glass per day. And finally, investigators at the Roswell Park Memorial Institute in New York and at Harvard University also describe a link between milk consumption and ovarian cancer.[128]

If this hypothesis is true, when we carry out human studies, we should find that women who have avoided meat throughout their lives will have a lower incidence of breast cancer. This is difficult to study in America, since there are few easily identifiable, large groups with such behavior patterns. The Seventh-Day Adventists are a religious group whose observing members avoid smoking and drinking. About half of them eat no meat. The rest eat some meat, but less than the general population. Studies show that the incidence of breast cancer is two and a half times greater among non-Adventist meat eaters than among the Adventist women. Vegetarian, non–Seventh-Day Adventist women also show a reduced level of breast cancer.[129] It is of interest that the vegetarians who consume eggs and milk (ovo-lacto vegetarians) have more breast cancer than the strict vegetarians (vegans) who eat nothing that comes from animals. Studies linking fat with breast cancer show a positive relationship with intake of animal fat, and animal protein, but *not* with plant fat.

The largest study on the relationship between meat intake and breast cancer comes from Japan. Dr. Takeshi Hirayama has been following a group of 122,000 people for many years. Women in this group who consumed meat seven or more times each week had a nearly four times greater chance (relative risk .83) of developing breast cancer compared with women eating no meat at all or just one time per week. Those with an intermediate usage (two to four times per week) were 2.55 times more likely to develop breast cancer than the low-usage group. Exactly the same trends developed for egg use. Butter and cheese also showed a similar pattern.[130] Plant-based diets protect against breast cancer. Animal-based diets predispose to breast cancer.

## Recommended Dietary Allowances

Most people argue that we need meat as a source of protein, but what does nutritional science tell us about the amount of protein needed for adults? The latest RDA (Recommended Dietary Allowances, tenth edition, 1989) produced by the National Research Council informs us of the recommended allowance for protein in a simple formula. It is 0.75 grams per kilogram of body weight per day. *This is a very small amount of protein.* For a woman weighing 140 pounds this computes to less than forty-eight grams of protein daily. (The average American woman eats about a hundred grams or more daily.) The forty-eight grams amount to about one and a half ounces, an amount that would easily fit in the lightly cupped palm of your hand. The World Health Organization (WHO) places the figure even lower at 0.6 g/kilo/day. This is only thirty-eight grams of protein, just a little over one ounce. Compare that with the usual eight-to-sixteen ounce steak served in America.

It is important to remember that protein does not have to originate from animal sources. Proteins from plant sources (for example, beans) are equivalent in quality to those from animal sources. Further, they are not contaminated with saturated fat, cholesterol, hormones, bacteria, viruses, pesticides, and the other harmful substances listed above. A surface coating of pesticides does not pose the same risk as pesticides concentrated within the food itself. Of course, all food should be properly washed. For those purely medical reasons, I feel plant sources of protein are preferable from a health standpoint. Stated another way, it is very difficult to fashion a health-supporting diet that includes the large amounts of meat and dairy products currently favored in America. We will not discuss the high cost of meat or the extremely large amounts of energy, feed, water, and fuel required to bring meat to the dining table, but these are very important considerations for our entire society.

There is no doubt that cardiovascular health is undermined by meat and dairy products, and there is also a great deal of evidence that cancer formation is also promoted by their use. Available animal experiments support this association.

## Think Before You Eat

If you choose to eat meat, I would first recommend sticking to the RDA amounts listed above. This eliminates the ingestion of huge portions of roast beef or large steaks. Then I would recommend using small amounts of fish or lean fowl because of the lessened amount of saturated fat compared with beef, pork, and lamb. Surprisingly, the amounts of cholesterol are almost identical in all meats; it is the saturated fat levels that are widely divergent. Among the methods of preparation, deep-fat frying is the worst, panfrying and charcoal broiling are slightly better. Baking is next best and the very best is steaming or poaching. For chicken, skinning does slightly reduce the amount of fat. Lean white meat of turkey and skinless chicken as well as very lean beef can be chosen from the land animals. Of the various flesh proteins, on balance, that found in deep-water fish is probably the least harmful. Some of the safest seafoods are abalone, cod, crab, Dover and English sole, halibut, marlin, red snapper, Pacific salmon, sand dabs, scallops, sea bass, sole, trout, and tuna.

In addition to our meat supply, we are confronted with a vast array of artificial foods. We are not adapted to chemically altered, commercial products. The human body may eventually adapt to test-tube, chemical "designer foods" created for prolonged shelf life in a store for "improved taste" or for other economic considerations. **And then again, it may not.**

I think that we will look back at this era in human nutrition as a time in which we experimented with nature's design and failed. We are creating an avalanche of heart disease, stroke, cancer, degenerative arthritis, obesity, and many other ills.

As far as breast cancer is concerned, the effect of our

rich American diet is undeniable. Is it sufficient, then, to change our eating habits alone if we wish to avoid breast cancer? Not quite, but almost. While diet is the most significant factor, there is another component of a breast-cancer-prevention plan—exercise.

# 8

## *The Exercise Factor*

*T*hus far we have stressed the crucial importance of diet in the prevention of breast cancer. Diet is the most important component of breast cancer prevention, but exercise is the other. Why is exercise protective? Because, like diet, exercise can affect not only overall health, but hormone activity as well.

The first doctor to call attention to the link between exercise and cancer was one of America's first cancer researchers, James Ewing. The year? 1911. He noted that the "well-to-do and indolent" were more likely to develop cancer than the "poor and overworked," and he related that protection to physical exertion. Unfortunately, few listened to him in an era when exercise was often equated with lowered economic status and a lower social class. From that time until the 1960s, most doctors advised their patients that excessive exercise would "wear out their bodies."

Now we know that exercise is associated not only with increased cardiovascular fitness and a lessened rate of heart attacks, but also with the reduction in numbers of several malignancies. Breast cancer is one of these, colon cancer is another. We also have evidence from Dr. Ralph Paffenbarger[131] that exercise provides an overall extension of life. In 1992, Paffenbarger confirmed his earlier 1975 findings in a Stanford University study.[132] In another large and well-designed study of exercise, heart disease, stroke, and cancer, reported in the *Journal of the American Medical Association*,[133] Steven Blair found that cancer deaths were nearly five times more common among the least fit of the 13,000 men and women studied. Another researcher[134] found that physical fitness and physical activity reduced breast cancer mortality as well as colon and prostate deaths. He postulated an effect on hormone metabolism (estrogen and prostaglandin).

At the Ontario Cancer Institute in Toronto, N. F. Boyd[135] also found a link between exercise and a reduced risk of breast cancer. Dr. Boyd confirmed that breast cancer patients can improve their prognosis by switching to a low-fat diet even after the diagnosis and treatment phase.

The National Health and Nutrition Examination Survey and a follow-up study examined the health of 7,407 women from 1971 until 1984. An increased risk of all cancer among inactive individuals was found. Specifically, the relative risk for breast cancer among inactive postmenopausal women was 1.7 times that for physically active persons. Adjustments were made for cigarette smoking, body weight, and other potential confounders.[136] Rose Frisch, Ph.D., at the Harvard School of Public Health, has written extensively on the relationship between exercise for women and their risk of cancer. She has consistently found that exercise protects against breast cancer, and postulates that this is because exercise reduces body fat. The *hydroxylation of estradiol* takes place in the body's fat. This complex process converts estradiol into a nonestrogenic substance, 2-OHE1, which is not a cancer promoter. The production of 2-OHE1 is increased with decreasing amounts of body fat.[137] Once again, the final pathway of breast cancer prevention is mediated by an alteration in hormone levels.

In 1985, Dr. Frisch studied 5,398 college graduates, half of whom were athletic, half of whom were not. The exercisers were not highly conditioned athletes. They simply started exercising before or during high school and continued this pattern into adulthood. *The nonathletic women were twice as likely to develop breast cancer.*[138] The protective features of exercise were even found to overcome other risk factors. In a follow-up study, also on athletes, Dr. Frisch found that the leaner women produced an inactive form of estrogen. The leaner athletes were often not lighter—muscle is heavy—however, they did have up to one-third less body fat. Muscle tissue not only is heavier than fatty tissue, but it also has a much **higher metabolic rate**: it burns calories faster and more efficiently than other bodily tissues. The overall metabolic rate of the human body is elevated by exercise and remains elevated for twelve to fifteen hours after an exercise session. Dr. Frisch and her coworkers also learned that former athletes were less likely to develop a wide variety of cancers—not just reproductive organ cancers.[139]

How can exercise reduce the probability of breast cancer? Exercise not only alters hormone levels in the body, it also enhances immune system function.[140] Natural killer (NK) cells are white blood cells that have a role in our defense against viruses, bacteria, and cancer. These NK cells increase in both numbers and activity during strenuous exercise or even with walking.[141] Similarly, immunoglobulins, tumor necrosis factor, interferons, and interleukins and other protective substances are released by exercise.[142] Leonard Cohen has been an important contributor to the scientific literature concerning the effect of diet on the formation of cancer in both humans and animals.[143] In one of his studies, four groups of rats were given breast cancer by administration of a chemical (nitrosomethylurea or NMU). The first group was placed on a low-fat diet, the second group on a medium-fat diet, and the third and fourth groups were both on a high-fat diet. In addition, the fourth group was given free access to an exercise wheel. The animals in the fourth group "ran" 1 to 2.8 miles per day, consumed more food, and even gained more weight than the sedentary rats. But they also had far less tumor growth as well as a longer period of time before the appearance of any tumor. The protective effect of regular exercise seemed to be more potent than the effect of a low-fat diet alone in this animal study. Human experience does not entirely support such a dramatic benefit for exercise, but we have learned that such well-conducted animal experiments should be carefully considered.

Exercise as rehabilitation following cancer treatment was investigated by three different groups widely spread over the country. All reported a positive impact on speed of recovery and quality of life. Even for patients receiving chemotherapy for breast cancer, aerobic exercise helped combat the usual weight gain.[144]

A study by John Vena, from the State University of New York at Buffalo, focused on women's cancers and also showed that substantial protection from breast cancer resulted from exercise.[145] These health benefits do not seem to require a tremendous amount of exercise. Modest but consistent efforts are very effective.

Aside from increasing the metabolic rate, endurance, and strength as well as improving digestion, exercise has profound mental effects. Advantages include an improved mood, and a sense of increased optimism and enthusiasm: these mental benefits make it easier for the exerciser to follow other dietary practices that are of even greater value. Regular exercisers also rarely suffer depression. It is unusual for a woman who has invested a good deal of physical, and even psychic, energy in a workout session to immediately "blow it" on capricious fatty-food indulgence. The effects of exercise not only include a firming of the muscles and an increase in endurance, but also increases in flexibility and coordination. (The latter is not a trivial advantage. Falls are a major source of injury and death in persons over 70 years of age.)

To illustrate the profound hormonal effects of prolonged strenuous exercise, it has been long known that among women who are serious marathon runners, a complete cessation of menstruation is common. It is less well-known that women who are extreme exercisers (marathon competitors, for example) and who allow this condition to persist for many years can actually develop osteoporosis. This is thought to result chiefly from very low estrogen levels. This negative effect is mentioned only to show that profound estrogen reduction can be achieved through maximal exertion. The incidence of amenorrhea (lack of menstrual periods) in premenopausal women in the United States has been reported to be between 2 and 5 percent, but the rate is from 4 to 66 percent of female athletes.

Thus, a *proper* amount of physical activity, especially during adolescence, is a nonhormonal method of reducing exposure to estrogen. This is accomplished, researchers believe, by the known effect of not only reducing the level of hormones in the body but also by reducing the total number of ovulatory menstrual cycles during a woman's reproductive life.

There is no doubt that our ancient ancestors were active, strong, and vigorous people. We know this from their skeletal remains, which clearly demonstrate robust and strong bones. More importantly, there were prominent and highly developed sites of attachment of muscles and tendons to those bones. This tells us that those muscles were large, and that our ancestors were much stronger than today's humans. The sedentary American lifestyle is a dangerous and recent aberration of behavior. Physical exercise is not only a tonic for the mind and mood, it is essential to keep our muscles, joints, and heart in good condition. The bonus is the reduction in the rate of breast cancer. You may want to make changes in your lifestyle, but wonder if it's too late. Is there a cutoff period, beyond which it is not possible to influence the development or the course of breast cancer? The answer is an unequivocal no. It's *never* too late to start.

# 9

## It's Never Too Late to Start

*I*t is always preferable to make beneficial changes early in life. But what about the women who only discover these prevention facts while in their sixties or seventies? Are they simply out of luck?

The totality of evidence suggests that meaningful dietary change can be helpful no matter when it takes place. A woman can benefit whether she changes her diet during early womanhood, the reproductive years, in early or late menopause, or even after the diagnosis of breast cancer has been made. The earlier such changes are made, the better. There appear to be two phases to the manipulation of breast cancer by dietary means. One is the primary prevention of the disease, and the other is the secondary retardation of the disease after the cancer is already established.

For a long while there was no credible, scientifically verifiable information on the point at which a good diet ceased to be effective. We were left with only the knowledge that breast cancer patients, matched for stage of disease, survived longer in those countries where low-fat diets were the norm, regardless of their age.[146]

The picture was finally clarified in an important and

unique 1993 Swedish study reporting on the beneficial effects of a low-fat diet for patients already diagnosed and treated for breast cancer with conventional therapies. The Swedish group, led by Lars-Erik Holm, found a 20-percent lessening of breast cancer recurrence in only forty-eight months on a low-fat diet, which equaled 12.4 percent of total calories.[147] Of interest was the observation that intermediate levels of fat intake had intermediate levels of protection, while the highest levels of breast cancer recurrence occurred in patients with the highest levels of fat and the lowest levels of fiber intake.

A prominent Canadian breast cancer researcher, Norman F. Boyd, also found a similar pattern of lessened disease recurrence in women eating a low-fat diet. In an editorial in the same issue of the *Journal of the National Cancer Institute* in which Holm's article appeared, he reviewed the relevant studies in the world's scientific literature and agreed with Holm's findings, concluding: "In addition to possible early effects on the development of breast cancer, fat also appears to have late effects, as might be expected of a promoter. This finding makes it more likely that interventions with dietary fat directed at the prevention of breast cancer in mid-life will be effective."[148]

David Gregorio and his associates from the Roswell Park Memorial Institute in New York also studied 953 women who had already been treated for breast cancer. These women were followed up for more than twelve years. The researchers found that the relative risk of death increased 44 percent for each thousand grams of fat consumed per month![149] Once again, here is dramatic proof from a rarely quoted and unusual study, that *fat fuels breast cancer*. It also teaches us that it is not too late to change one's diet even after the diagnosis of breast cancer has been made. The Roswell Park study concluded that lowering your fat intake can increase your life span if you have had breast cancer treatment.

These studies are very significant. There have been previous similar reports, but the matter was never so conclusively demonstrated with properly performed, randomized studies. Remember, the subjects were women who made dietary changes *after* they were diagnosed with breast cancer.

One of the first modern reports of hormone changes in response to diet was based on a small group of postmenopausal breast cancer patients studied in 1984 by Dr. John A. McDougall, then of Hawaii. His short-term study documented remarkable drops in prolactin levels (38 percent), total estrogen (36.6 percent), and estradiol (45 percent) in response to an 8-percent-fat diet.[150] In preparing this chapter, I spoke to one of his original subjects from the 1984 study who continues to be in excellent health with no evidence of recurring breast cancer. Ruth Heidrich, Ph.D. has maintained the very same ultra-low-fat diet to the present and has no thoughts of ever changing back to the standard American diet with its 34 to 44 percent of calories from fat. Incidentally, she has completed seven grueling triathlons and over forty marathons despite her fifty-nine-plus years, and has written an excellent book—*A Race for Life: From Cancer to the Ironman*—relating her experiences.[151] She finds that her eating plan contributes to improved endurance compared with other athletes eating a "balanced American diet."

Variations on the timing issue come from Laval University in Quebec, Canada. René Verreault and his associates[152] focused on the diet during the year preceding the diagnosis of breast cancer. Those patients consuming the largest amount of fat had a nearly twofold greater incidence of axillary lymph-node involvement with tumor. That is the spread of breast cancer from the breast to the lymph glands in the underarm area, a phenomenon associated with a worsened prognosis. These Canadian researchers speculated that diet could have contributed to this condition in the following ways: by changing the hormonal profile (remember, prolonged high estrogen levels contribute to breast cancer), by directly promoting the growth of any breast cancer cells present, by altering the structure of cell membranes or hormone receptors in the cells, and by the process of converting secretions from the adrenal glands to estrogen in the body's fatty tissue. A second and similar study from Canada showed that breast cancer patients with greater body weight had shortened survival times.[153] Scientific work of this type is rarely done, but there is striking consistency in the existing data.

Women who live in countries with low-fat diets and who do develop breast cancer live longer than closely matched women in countries with high-fat diets. The five-year survival for Japanese breast cancer patients is 17.6 percent greater compared with matched patients from Boston, Massachusetts.

Let's examine three representative groups of women who might alter their diets and anticipate the probable effects.

First, young women. We have learned that dietary changes made early in life are more powerful than those made later. The totality of available evidence supports this conclusion. These young women should enjoy a markedly reduced risk of breast cancer. However, they will not be totally protected against breast cancer. There is no group of women anywhere in the world that is totally free of this disease, but they will be greatly protected by a low-fat and high-fiber diet. How much protection? The optimists estimate 80 percent, the pessimists estimate 60 percent, and the scoffers say none. Decide for yourself.

The next group of women would be those who, although older, do not have breast cancer. They should be substantially protected by the dietary measures I will describe, much as the young women above.

A third group would be women who have the beginnings of breast cancer that has not become clinically evident. If the tumor is in the early phases of its development, there is good, but indirect, evidence that it will be at least retarded in its growth by the removal of promoting factors. This is similar to the effect of depriving a weed of water, sun, and fertilizer. The weed is still alive, but not able to flourish. Can breast cancer be killed by depriving it of growth-promoting factors? I suspect so, but cannot cite evidence for this position. Further, I don't know how such an experiment could be established. We must accept that some matters simply cannot be tested.

For older women without the diagnosis of breast cancer, the effects of dietary change will be partially diluted by their age, but still very desirable. I have the experience of many of my older patients to report to you. In every case, they have experienced improvement in their overall health and feelings of well-being as well as contributing to their protection against breast cancer. I can think of no exception. An intangible benefit to such a woman is the knowledge that she is not a passive victim. She is actively contributing to her own care. Remember that heart disease and stroke are more likely, on a statistical basis alone, to take an older woman's life. The probabilities of these conditions are substantially reduced by the dietary measures we are recommending.

The final group would include those women who already have diagnosed breast cancer. We formerly had no proof that a dietary change at that late stage would be of help, although I recommended it on an empirical basis. I thought it would be helpful, and it's always better to be in the best health possible when combating a serious disease. It now seems that such thinking was much too timid. Thanks to the Swedish, Canadian, and other[154, 155] studies mentioned earlier, I can tell you that scientific evidence strongly supports the value of change. Total survival, as well as disease-free intervals, were both significantly extended. This is also being confirmed in animal studies. Dr. Gary Meadows of Washington State University[156] found that animals given cancers (in this case, melanoma) were substantially protected from tumor growth by the restriction of protein (specifically, two amino acids, phenylalanine and tyrosine). Meadows can envision a time when physicians will prescribe a specific diet as an addition to standard therapies. That is exactly what we are advocating in this book.

When you look critically at the totality of the scientifically respectable data, your conclusion will be the same as mine: *it's never too late to change!*

# The Breast-Cancer-Prevention Food Plan

W hat follows is a *plan for eating, not a diet.* In most diets, food portions are measured, weighed, counted, or otherwise limited. *In this plan, portions are not limited.* The food in this plan is based on starchy plants, vegetables, and fruit. It is simplicity itself. You should always eat to satisfaction. Any eating plan that leaves you chronically hungry and depending on self-control to keep from eating more will fail.

Recommended foods include potatoes, rice, corn, beans, whole grains, breads, egg-free pastas, and all vegetables and fruits. These are delicious, familiar, inexpensive, and easily available. Particularly important are the three groups of foods that inhibit cancer: first, the *protease inhibitors* soybeans, chickpeas, lentils, limas, and red, black, and white beans; second, *cruciferous vegetables* including broccoli, Brussels sprouts, cabbage, and cauliflower; and third, the *beta-carotenes*, including carrots, yams, sweet potatoes, tomatoes, green leafy vegetables, squash, pumpkin, apricots, spinach, asparagus, broccoli, deep green lettuce, and cantaloupe. Highly pigmented foods—green, yellow, orange, and red—all have protective qualities. Simply use your eyes; you don't need a chart. These foods also add vitamins, minerals, and fiber. Nuts and seeds are used in small amounts due to their high-fat content; however, this small amount is desirable for the essential fatty acids and vitamin E, both of which can act as cancer-fighting antioxidants.

Can the value of such a simple plan be scientifically defended? The researchers at the National Cancer Institute have completed a massive survey of the world's scientific literature on the subject of vegetable and fruit consumption and cancer incidence.[157] They reviewed a total of 156 studies. Of these, 128 noted protection from cancer provided by the vegetables and fruits. Groups with the lowest fruit-and-vegetable consumption had twice the overall rate of cancer.

Animal proteins are minimized or eliminated in this plan. If you feel that you need some animal protein, the safest is deep-saltwater fish. If animal protein is used, it is preferable to use it as a flavoring, garnish, or as an accent rather than as a main course. The meat-centered American meal should be a thing of the past.

Note that our health-promoting meal plan is centered on starchy plants (complex carbohydrates), vegetables, leafy plants, and fruit rather than meat and dairy products. Young people often express concerns about lack of strength on a low-meat or nonmeat diet. This is unfounded. Numerous scientific studies show increases of strength, and particularly endurance, on this eating plan. The Hawaii Ironman Triathlon is probably the most strenuous athletic test of endurance on record. *Vegetarians have dominated the event for years.* Meat eaters simply run out of muscle glycogen; athletes call this *running into the wall.* Athletes now identify the vegetarian diet as "carbo-loading." (Carl Lewis, the great American sprinter, follows this meal plan. One of his favorite techniques when he has to eat in a restaurant is to eat *two* typical American dinners, but minus the meat portions.[158]

I discourage all use of cow's milk and all other dairy products, even including nonfat milk, yogurt, and cheese. Is this unduly strict? or even radical? Let's not simply accept the use of dairy products as a "given." Although dairy products have become a central part of our food culture, and many of us have come to prefer their taste, the only health-oriented reason to use them is for their calcium and protein contents. Calcium, however, is much more safely and completely obtained from foods grown in the earth—after all, that's where the cow gets it! In fact, it's difficult to design a diet that is deficient in calcium when there are sufficient calories to meet daily needs.

Did you know that human beings are the only mammals on earth that continue to drink milk after weaning? Not only that, but we drink the milk of another species of mammal. We also induce some of our domesticated animals to do the same. Despite the fact that milk drinking is widespread among Westernized people, it truly is a bizarre habit.

Drinking nonfat milk does not solve the problem, since the protein and milk-sugar portions of the milk are even further concentrated when the fat is removed. For example, with skim milk, the lactose (milk sugar) fraction is 57 percent. It is only 30 percent in whole milk. Allergic reactions are more likely with nonfat milk due to the increased protein fraction. The hazard of osteoporosis in adults and diabetes in children is made worse by the use of skim milk compared with whole milk, due to the very heavy protein load. Most American women eat far too much protein; they certainly don't need any more.

Finally, in this eating plan, fats are avoided when possible. Oils are used only in trace amounts or sparingly at most. If oil *must* be used, use olive oil. Avoid hydrogenated oils and vegetable oils such as corn oil, soybean oil, and safflower-seed oil. Omega-3 oils and certain omega-6 oils are permissible in small amounts. Eggs are avoided, or minimized. No margarine, butter, or dairy-based cheeses are included. Soy-based cheeses can be used occasionally (some are available with reduced or no fat).

Let's talk about the V-word—vegetarianism! When first hearing of this eating plan, my patients will often look at me with a look combining horror and pity and exclaim, "Are you a vegetarian?" My answer is, "Not always, but I'm trying to be." Not all vegetarians eat well, and some vegetarians eat a diet that is downright dangerous. For example, I live near a prominent gourmet vegetarian restaurant. Their cuisine can be loaded with butter, cheese, cream, nuts, oils, eggs, and mayonnaise. A trip to this wonderful place leaves me feeling stuffed and sick—but the food is widely regarded as health-promoting.

One of my colleagues tells of a medical-school classmate who didn't want to harm animals and became a vegetarian on an ethical, not a health, basis. His notion of a "vegetarian lunch" was a bag of potato chips and a Coke. Simply not eating meat isn't enough.

Some people even consider themselves vegetarians if they exclude only red meat. A much larger group are the ovo-lacto vegetarians who use milk, dairy products, and eggs, but no meat, fish, or poultry. Presumably they also use added oils. The only vegetarians whose actions truly make sense to me are the vegans (pronounced "*vee*-guns"). Vegans avoid all animal products including meat, milk, milk products, eggs, and sometimes even honey. They may use added oils, though the more informed use only trifling amounts. If added oils are used, they should be the monounsaturated oils (olive), or certain omega-3 and -6 oils as mentioned above.

My personal approach is based more on health considerations than on ethical or moral ones. (This fits with American vegetarians in general, with only 24 percent of them becoming so for ethical, animal welfare, and environmental reasons combined.) But I will admit immediately that if called upon to approach a cow and kill, bleed, skin, and dehoof it, chainsaw its carcass, cut the muscle from the bones, dispose of the bones, joints, intestines, intestinal contents, tendons, stomach, blood, and lungs, then heat the remaining chunks of muscle over a fire prior to putting them in my mouth and chewing—I would become a very strict vegetarian immediately.

What is the relationship between protein and the health of our bones? Few people realize that *excessive protein intake is a major contributor to osteoporosis.* Here is how it happens. When protein is eaten in marked excess of daily requirements, most of that excess must be promptly excreted in the urine as amino acids. (Proteins are composed of amino acids.) As the sulfur-containing amino acids from meat are eliminated, they cause a strongly acidic condition. This creates a need for a great deal of neutralizing material called cation. This is where calcium comes into the picture. It is necessary to balance the acidic condition. As the acid is eliminated, a severe load is placed on the kidneys and is accompanied by large losses of calcium. As there is very little calcium in the blood, the calcium is drawn out of the bones. These calcium losses are particularly important when you realize that high levels of protein ingestion will place you in a negative calcium balance, regardless of calcium intake or hormone intake.

When this condition is maintained over many years, the result is osteoporosis. Osteoporosis is prevalent in precisely those countries where the most milk, calcium pills, and estrogen tablets are used. Compare this with the near absence of osteoporosis in countries with no milk, no calcium pills, and no estrogen tablets! Excessive protein intake accompanies lifelong negative calcium balances. Despite profit-motivated messages from the milk industry who claim that their product is essential.

There is no shortage of information on the relationship

between excess protein intake and osteoporosis. This information has been available in the scientific literature on physiology since 1910! I have 141 references from peer-reviewed journals in my files. Yet the medical establishment is just becoming aware of this long-documented problem. In a study from Yale University School of Medicine, attention was directed to thirty-four published studies from sixteen countries. Dietary calcium or total caloric intake could not plausibly explain the age-adjusted hip-fracture incidence in industrialized countries. The authors agree that the elevated acid production associated with a high animal-protein diet might lead to chronic bone loss in order to supply calcium for the "buffering" of the excess acid. This, over years, would be easily responsible for bone dissolution, or osteoporosis.[159]

Protein does not have to originate from animal sources. Many nutritionists and nutritional charts underestimate the contribution that vegetables make to your daily protein requirements. Despite what you may have been told, plant protein is of high quality. It carries with it none of the problems of cholesterol, saturated fat, and contamination with bacteria, viruses, antibiotics, and hormones. Even the pesticide problem is greatly reduced. Pesticides, if they exist on plants and vegetables, can almost always be washed off. In meat, they are concentrated in the fatty tissue and are not removable. All of the essential amino acids are synthesized by plants. None are synthesized by animals. Many vegetables contain substantial amounts of protein, from three to over eight grams per cup, including: peas, kale, Brussels sprouts, broccoli, sweet potatoes, and asparagus. Grains are also an excellent source of protein, as are pasta, oatmeal, brown rice, and whole-wheat bread. Over two thirds of all humans on this planet satisfy the great majority of their protein needs from plant sources. To use mostly animal sources for protein is a practice that only the very wealthiest nations can indulge. Dr. T. Colin Campbell, in his huge study of Chinese dietary practices (the "Cornell-China Study"), found that the Chinese derived only 11 percent of their protein from animal sources. Americans, by contrast, typically obtain more than 70 percent of their protein from animal sources! Wherever you look around the world, there is a striking positive correlation between the amount of ingested animal foods and rates of cancer, heart disease, and osteoporosis. This is not a coincidence.

You should also be aware that animal-protein intake well above the RDA has been consistently linked with increases in the rates of several cancers. It is difficult to distinguish between the contribution of animal **protein** and the effect of the **fat** associated with that protein. There seems to be a consistent and profound association between cancer and large amounts of animal protein.[160, 161] We must also remember that we do not eat the same meat as our ancient ancestors did. We eat artificially fattened, hormonally treated, obese, and often ill animals.

## The Plan at a Glance

• Reduce your dietary fat intake to *no more than* 20 percent of total calories. The optimum goal is 10 percent.

• Base your diet on rice, potatoes, corn, beans, whole grains, and pasta. These are foods that grow from the ground.

• Eat lots of fresh vegetables and fruit. Stress the cancer-fighting foods listed earlier.

• Eat plenty of fiber. (The average American eats a mere eleven grams of fiber a day—this should at least be doubled, but thirty or even thirty-five grams is best.)

• Avoid dairy products.

• Minimize or avoid animal protein.

• Minimize or avoid alcohol.

• Water is the ideal beverage.

- Avoid oils.
- I recommend vitamin supplements. In addition to a good multiple-vitamin preparation, include additional vitamins E, C, and beta-carotene. Although this subject is hotly debated, I believe that the balance of evidence favors the use of these antioxidant vitamins. The subject of correct dosage is also contested and I will simply give you my daily doses: Vitamin C in the one-to-three-gram range, vitamin E, four hundred to eight hundred international units, and 25,000 I.U.s of beta-carotene per day. Some authorities feel that even greater amounts are preferable for cancer prevention.

That's it! The plan is simple and straightforward, but its lifesaving benefits are inestimable. The plan should not only reduce breast cancer risk, but can also substantially reduce the risk of nearly all the other big killers in American life: heart disease, stroke, other cancers, hypertension, and diabetes. We know that this dietary plan is safe. Nearly all of the humans who have ever lived on this earth, over a span of millions of years, have proven it.

Although the plan may sound severe, I assure you that motivated people adapt to it easily. The benefits in energy and feeling of well-being are remarkable and immediate, while the long-term gains are an added bonus.

Don't depend on doctors, scientists, or the government for guidance. You must protect yourself and take action on your own behalf. This is the essence of empowerment for women. Women want choices and control, not breast cancer.

In particular, please don't depend on breast surgeons (such as myself), oncologists, radiologists, and radiotherapists to rescue you from breast cancer. Although we do the best we can, we are only successful in the treatment of a percentage of cases, and then usually because the disease happened to be detected in a favorable stage. The majority of us are not oriented toward prevention, and we are not miracle workers; we simply do what we can. Too often we are not happy with the outcome. I realize that many health professionals will not accept this paragraph with good grace. Let me say that I am not denigrating their efforts, or mine, in behalf of our patients. Breast cancer is devastating and best avoided. Extensive studies provided by the National Surgical Adjuvant Breast Project show no significant increased survival rate for a particular surgical approach.

Breast cancer is a disease that is best to prevent instead of treat. You can "be scientific" and wait fifteen or more years for a "definitive" study to be completed, or you can act now on the evidence currently available to you. *Continue your efforts at early detection*, but why not begin protecting yourself and your family now through preventive measures.

Medical authorities all too often tell you that a complex disease like breast cancer is beyond your control and that only "experts" can properly give advice and suggest treatment. I don't believe this. I believe that women can examine the available evidence, make personal decisions, and acquire the knowledge and skill to help themselves. If they act with this knowledge, they are likely not to be among the one of seven women some experts feel will develop breast cancer by the end of this decade.

I'm often asked about "cheating" on the diet plan. How strict should one be? I believe one should be as careful as possible. Even relatively small amounts of fat ingested daily and over a long time span can do very large amounts of damage. I feel that the evidence concerning the hydrogenated fats is particularly damning—these fats are more like chemicals than foods. When you eat a modern food that contains substantial amounts of hydrogenated fats, within minutes, molecules of those fats are coursing through the capillaries of your body and either entering or surrounding each of the several trillion cells within your body. (The only exceptions are the hardest parts of your teeth, your hair, and your fingernails.) There could be no closer or more profoundly intimate association with your food environment. Only you have control over the most important environment of all, the interior of your body.

But the real reason for making these changes is to enjoy more holiday seasons with the people you love, to be around when the grandchildren get married—and perhaps to be there to teach your great-granddaughters and nieces how to avoid breast cancer, too.

# Getting Started: Sample Meal Plans

*D*oes the breast-cancer-prevention diet contain huge amounts of foods like "tempeh" and "tamari"? The answer is no. Can it be followed by an average American woman? The answer is yes. Most of the foods are common, inexpensive items available in any local supermarket. It is not necessary to shop at a health food store or a special market. However, you may find a broader range of nonfat, whole-grain breads, grains, and other useful products in health food stores. Remember, this eating plan is based on *good foods that grow in the ground.* That simple phrase will help you if confusion sets in.

Let's start with a single day's food; then we'll expand it to a week.

## A Break from Tradition

A *rich American breakfast* might include orange juice, fried eggs, bacon, ham or sausage, oil-fried hash-brown potatoes, white toast with butter or margarine, coffee with cream and sugar, and maybe a sweet roll. This high-fat, high-cholesterol, low-fiber meal might be tasty, but does not support health. About 65 percent of the calories in this breakfast come from fat and oil!

By contrast, a *breakfast to promote health* and diminish the chance of breast cancer might include the following: a very large serving (or even two) of an easy-to-cook cereal—oatmeal, oat bran, or other grain cereal—cooked with a touch of vanilla and water, to avoid the need for milk. Fruit such as peaches, apricots, dates, or bananas may be added for sweetness and flavor. If sugar is desired, it is sprinkled on the surface, not mixed throughout the cereal. This maximizes the sweetness and minimizes the total sugar load. Sugar represents "empty calories," but its use is unrelated to breast cancer. Whole-grain, oil-free nonfat toast, with fruit preserves or jam, and fresh cantaloupe could follow. This delicious and filling breakfast contains a trifling 6 to 8 percent of calories from fat. If cold cereal is preferred, choose a non-sugared variety without added oils, and wherever possible, use nonfat soy milk or rice milk instead of cow's milk.

Not only is it not a burden to eat this way, but many meals are easier and cheaper to prepare. You will *immediately* feel better as a bonus. Become a "label detective." Examine in detail the labels on the foods that you buy. Avoid those with fat, oil, eggs, milk products, and especially hydrogenated fats and oils.

## Other Breakfast Tips

Don't skip breakfast. Skipping this meal will lower your metabolic rate and make you ravenously hungry later in the day. The most obese people in our country typically skip breakfast, have a light lunch, but indulge in a large high-fat, main meal in the evening—often just before retiring. Don't fall into this trap; it could defeat your eating plan.

When you're in a hurry, don't stop off at a fast-food place. Most of their breakfasts average a disastrous 40 to 50 percent of calories as fat. Doughnuts, croissants, and rolls are all fat-laden, as are eggs, sausages, bacon, and ham. Even the allegedly healthy bran muffins are usually very high in fat. A quick breakfast could be a piece of fruit and a sugar-less, whole grain cereal or oatmeal. When possible, avoid granulated sugar or artificial sweeteners; they're not "poison," but they're not good for you either. Bagels are usually fat-free; use apple butter instead of cream cheese.

I also don't recommend the traditional orange juice. I know, I know! You've been told all your life that juices are good for you. But I have the following reservations concerning concentrated juices. They are often sugar-laden, which will give your serum insulin level a sharp elevation, and they have no fiber or "filling" qualities. Eat the whole fruit—it's better in every way. Drink water with each meal, and in between as well.

Breakfasts are wonderful meals for women who want to reduce their risk of breast cancer.

For those occasions when more time is available, steel-cut or Irish oatmeals, whole-grain pancakes, waffles, or French toast made with egg whites and the smallest amount of oil possible, are health-supporting and a delicious change. Use a Teflon pan with a small amount of nonstick spray. Serve with fresh fruit, no-sugar-added jams, apple butter, or a small amount of maple syrup.

## Lean Lunching

Let's contrast a high-fat, low-fiber lunch with a health-promoting lunch. A *typical American lunch* might include a double hamburger with cheese, french-fried potatoes, and a malt or cola beverage. Once again, this meal would be very high in fat (about 55 percent of calories) and low in fiber.

A *health-promoting lunch* might include a salad with a vinegar dressing or a nonfat, noncholesterol dressing. The main dish could be two complex carbohydrates (such as new potatoes and sweet corn) and a vegetable. Whole-grain bread with preserves for a spread can be added if desired. For dessert, have fruit. This lunch contains less than 10 percent of calories from fat.

If you pack your own lunch, you might save some of your dinner portion from the night before. For lunch you can enjoy one of many variations of raw-vegetable salads. For dressing use balsamic vinegar, rice vinegar, plain vinegar, or a squeeze of lemon. Nonfat, noncholesterol dressings are also fine. The goal with salad dressings is to eliminate fat, oil, and salt as far as possible. Chef's salad is also permissible in our eating plan, but without the hard-boiled egg and cheeses. Leave off the ham, too; just increase the other ingredients. Tuna salad for the meat eaters is all right if the tuna is water-packed. Don't add regular mayonnaise, though. Small quantities of the new nonfat, noncholesterol mayonnaises are worth a try. Spinach salad is fine without bacon—try substituting apple slices and raisins. Commercial pasta salads are usually drenched in oil, so avoid them or make your own.

Dressings are the biggest problem with the average salad. Thousand island, blue cheese, ranch, and other dressings are incredibly high in fat. Don't even think of them! Even the "low-cal" or "light" Italian variety is usually extremely high in added oils. Use balsamic vinegar or other vinegars, lemon juice, salsa or red cocktail sauce, or nonfat, noncholesterol dressings instead. You will learn to really taste the vegetables again instead of a greasy dressing that masks real flavor and will torpedo your eating plan!

Here is a tip for the use of even a fairly rich salad dressing as long as it is not too thick. First, toss the entire salad with your favorite dressing. Then spin the salad in a "spinner" used to dry lettuce after rinsing. This will leave only a very thin layer of dressing evenly coated on all the salad ingredients. If you're eating at a salad bar, you will have a wide variety of choices. Head for the broccoli, carrots, chickpeas or garbanzos (remember, they're among the cancer-canceling protease inhibitors), lettuce, peas, mushrooms, tomatoes, and cucumbers. Eliminate bacon, cheeses, eggs, rich salad dressings, oily premixed pasta salads, potato salads, and macaroni salads with mayonnaise. Most salad bars offer several vinegars to sprinkle on your salad.

Soups can make up a large category of delicious lunch items. These are vegetable, minestrone, noodle, bean, onion, and tomato or broth-based soups. They should not include cream, excessive added fat, meat, or cheese. If small amounts of meat are desired for flavoring or accent, this is optional. You may not be aware that there are ways of creating a creamy soup without cream. For example, a creamy mushroom soup can be made by cooking chopped mushrooms and pearl barley with vegetable stock (defatted chicken broth if desired), onions, garlic, and sherry. After forty minutes, puree the soup in batches, and recombine with added coarsely chopped cooked mushrooms for "mouth feel" and texture. Add spices to taste. Cornstarch can also be used as a thickening agent in soups, vegetable stews, and sauces.

The same approach is possible with tomato soup using rice as an expander. Carrot soup with rice and curry is another excellent substitute for a cream soup. My favorite is potato-leek soup made using the above techniques. In addition to the chunks of potato, the pureed potato gives a thick creamy mouth-feel and consistency. Garlic, cilantro, and other spices are added to taste. All of these soups feel and taste rich, but they are exceptionally low in fat and remarkably delicious.

Nonfat soups are available in supermarkets and specialty stores. They are either canned or packaged dry in paper containers. Keep some on hand for situations when you are short of time.

Sandwiches are a mainstay of American lunches. The traditional American hamburger is a poor choice with its high saturated fat and cholesterol levels. Mayonnaise—at 99 percent fat—is also off the list as an acceptable ingredient. Grilled cheese is also high in fat and cholesterol. Forget the egg sandwiches, too. Vegetable sandwiches, however, can be terrific—they are filling and virtually fat free. Use a whole-grain, non-oil bread and add sprouts, tomatoes, lettuce, mustard, and onions, if desired. If you must have a bit more fat or animal protein, you can use avocado or small amounts of lean turkey breast. For the tuna enthusiasts, use modest amounts, making sure that it's water-packed. Healthful breads include many whole-grain varieties as well as pita bread, rye, pumpernickel, sourdough, and even corn tortillas. Read labels and select the most natural whole-grain, fat-free product. Sandwich fillings for vegetable sandwiches can include red and green bell peppers, sliced onions, scallions, spinach, cucumber slices, and sliced baked potatoes (try it, it's excellent). More complex fillings for sandwiches include mashed beans or mashed split peas or garbanzos in a pita pocket. I prefer small amounts of salsa as a condiment; mustard is another favorite. It may sound strange to think of a sandwich without meat, but try it—you'll find that the taste you like may have more to do with the condiments and bread!

If you have access to more formal entrées at lunch, steamed vegetable plates are perfect without added butter or cheese. I like combining one vegetable with two starches, say, mashed potatoes and sweet corn with asparagus. Baked potatoes are always fine, but be very careful what you put on them. Beans make a great potato topping. (For that matter they make a good entree.) Other quick toppings include ketchup, barbecue sauce, steak sauce, or low-fat soups.

If you think that you will have to give up gravies and sauces for the rest of your life, consider this. Vegetable stocks that can include small amounts of meat or broth can be reduced (or boiled down) to a saucelike or gravylike consistency. With the addition of herbs or spices—such as cilantro, garlic, oregano, or fresh parsley—a wonderful sauce is created. For additional body, add pureed potatoes or cornstarch, to give the "mouth feel" that is associated with fatty foods.

Make vegetable stocks by gently simmering a mix of vegetables in water for about a half hour to an hour with added spices, then straining it. Use one teaspoonful of sesame oil or less to gently sauté one cup of onions and a half cup each of sliced celery, leeks, carrots, mushrooms, and turnips or parsnips. Add three smashed cloves of garlic, and parsley, cilantro, peppercorns, cloves, thyme, and herbs in small amounts along with five cups of water. Use fresh herbs and spices if available—they enhance flavor.

After simmering, strain the mix and discard the solid material. The vegetable stock can be used immediately, or placed in plastic ice-cube trays and frozen for use up to six months later. This vegetable stock can be used as a substitute for oil: as a sauce, or as a gravy, as a soup base, or for sautéing. The addition of whisked-in cornstarch or pureed potatoes, rice, or pearl barley can create whatever consistency you desire, from a thin liquid to a near paste. Canned vegetable stock is also available in the soup section of many supermarkets.

## The Delights of Dinner

In the United States, a rich evening meal typically centers around animal protein—often a large broiled or fried steak. A small, waterlogged portion of vegetable and a "starch" such as buttered corn or mashed potatoes with gravy might be side dishes. Pie, cake, or ice cream round off the meal. Such a dinner has a fat content of 70 percent of total calories and a very low fiber content.

A cancer-preventing, health-supporting evening meal could be: appetizers of sliced raw carrots, celery sticks, turnips, and baked (nonfat) corn chips with salsa. Next, a soup—perhaps onion, potato–leek, or vegetable. The main course could be pasta with a marinara (tomato-based) sauce and two fresh vegetables selected from among the beta-carotenes, such as kale and carrots. Lean animal protein could be used in this meal but only as a flavoring, accent, or garnish in the pasta sauce instead of as the focus of the meal. A fruit salad or frozen sorbet makes a great dessert served with non-fat or low-fat cookies, such as gingersnaps. A leisurely dinner with delicious food and good companionship is one of the great pleasures in life. It doesn't have to shorten that life.

If you do not wish to avoid meats completely, there are several ways to reduce your meat consumption to a healthier level. First, choose smaller portions. A sixteen-ounce steak is unnecessary and unhealthy. Second, choose meats that have the lowest saturated fat content, such as white turkey meat or skinned chicken breast. Broiled or poached fish has the advantage of providing fats as omega-3 fats rather than more harmful varieties. Avoid frying, sautéing in oil, or barbecuing. Remember, you can live healthily without any animal flesh whatever.

### Snacks

What should you do when the "munchies" strike? In the old days, the situation was rather grim. Three ounces of potato chips, an average serving, can total as much as thirty-five grams of fat! Even a single ounce of corn chips can contain eight or nine grams of fat. The salt load in each is also excessive. It is exciting to see new, totally nonfat products emerging—nonfat pretzels and baked tortilla chips, as well as other tasty and healthful low-fat or nonfat snack foods. Some of these products are also salt-free. Even oven-roasted potato chips without fat are available. They actually taste like potatoes, not like salt and oil. One ounce of these has less than a hundred calories and essentially no fat. Read the labels carefully—some products claim to be fat-free but actually contain fat. As always, avoid hydrogenated oils. Pretzels and pretzel chips containing only flour, water, yeast, and salt are available. Hot-air-popped popcorn is a late-night favorite; don't add oil. I use a small amount of soy sauce tossed with the kernels to give a little salt flavor (regular salt will not stick to air-popped kernels). Chili powder or other powdered seasonings are other flavoring options. Note that this low-fat eating plan does not include portion control. You eat to satisfaction, not to a premeasured weight or volume of food. In our household, we keep small, crisp apples in the refrigerator, as well as a large plastic container of pared carrot and celery sticks, along with sliced turnips, cucumbers, and green or yellow peppers. These are important. When I return from a hard day's work and head toward the refrigerator for a snack, I don't know the meaning of the term self-control. The pre-prepared vegetable bowl saves the day. I usually supplement the vegetables with non-fat tortilla chips and salsa for an entirely satisfying snack that holds me until dinner. One of my patients boils a large supply of small new potatoes and keeps them in a plastic bag for munching at home or at work. Make healthy foods as easy to reach for as a disastrous candy bar, rich ice cream or cookies! Several national bakeries have introduced fat-free lines of cakes, cookies, and crackers. These products are not low in calories or sugar, but are fat-free, and are acceptable for an occasional treat.

## The Rest of the Week

Here are sample menus for the remainder of a typical week of a cancer prevention diet. Whenever possible, include the cancer-fighting foods: beans, cantaloupe, apricots, pink grapefruit, cabbage, cauliflower, broccoli, squashes, carrots, tomatoes, peppers and all kinds of leafy greens including romaine lettuce, chard, turnip greens, and parsley.

## Day 2

*Breakfast*
Whole-grain French toast made with egg whites and low-fat soy milk
Fruit spread or maple syrup
Fresh fruit

*Lunch*
Low-fat vegetable soup
Sliced tomato and cucumber salad with vinegar or nonfat dressing
Tuna sandwich, containing a small amount—perhaps one or two ounces—of water-packed tuna with nonfat mayonnaise, lettuce, tomatoes, and sprouts
Fruit for dessert

*Dinner*
Mixed green salad with rice vinegar
Bean enchiladas with salsa in corn tortillas
Spanish rice
Lemon pudding without egg yolks

## DAY 3

*Breakfast*
> Hash-brown potatoes cooked in a nonstick pan without oil; barbecue sauce or salsa on the side
> Whole-wheat toast with fruit spread
> Pink grapefruit

*Lunch*
> Mixed bean salad on lettuce
> Whole-grain bread or pita sandwich with lettuce, tomato, onion, sprouts, and humus spread
> Carrot, celery, and red pepper sticks

*Dinner*
> Navy-bean soup
> Garden salad with a nonfat dressing
> Noodles with mushrooms and a pureed tomato-and-garlic sauce
> Sliced fresh fruit or berries

## DAY 4

*Breakfast*
> Wheat-flour pancakes with fruit spread or apple butter
> Cantaloupe slices

*Lunch*
> Pastina soup
> Tostada, meatless or with slivers of chicken breast, lettuce, tomatoes, beans, salsa

Vegetable sticks
Banana

*Dinner*
Lentil soup
Coleslaw with nonfat mayonnaise
Poached fish with lemon slices and asparagus
Polenta
Sorbet

## DAY 5

*Breakfast*
Shredded wheat with rice milk or soy milk and fruit
Whole–wheat toast with orange marmalade

*Lunch*
Split-pea soup
"Veggie sandwich" on whole-grain bread or toast
Ear of corn
Mixed berries

*Dinner*
Bean salad
Pasta primavera with broccoli, onions, and cauliflower
Tapioca pudding or sorbet

## DAY 6

*Breakfast*
> Irish oatmeal (steel-cut oats) or regular oatmeal with fruit
> Whole-grain toast with strawberry preserves

*Lunch*
> Spinach salad
> Vegetable curry with whole-grain rice
> Apple

*Dinner*
> Garden salad
> Baked snapper with a spicy tomato sauce
> Oven-baked "french fries"
> Steamed summer squash
> Poached pears with raspberry sauce

## DAY 7

*Breakfast*
> Cold cereal with fruit and soy milk
> Whole-grain toast
> Cantaloupe

*Lunch*
> Pastina soup
> Niçoise salad with lettuce, boiled potatoes, red onions, tomatoes, a small amount of water-packed tuna if desired, lemon, and vinegar
> Banana

*Dinner*
    Minestrone (Italian vegetable soup)
    Tomato salad with chopped scallions and balsamic
        vinegar
    Low-fat risotto with asparagus
    Whole-wheat French bread
    Apricots or sliced peaches in season

There is a sample week. Remember, try to include cabbage, cauliflower, squash, and all kinds of greens such as
chard, turnip greens, kale, spinach, broccoli, and turnips.


## About Beverages

Rely heavily on water—*water is the absolutely essential
fluid that our human bodies are designed for*. The exception
is mother's milk for infants and newborns. Options include
any of the dozens of sparkling waters on the market. A
squeeze of lemon or lime, adds flavor and visual appeal. For
those wishing a warm beverage with meals, herbal teas or
roasted-grain beverages are fine.

Coffee in moderation is optional. While no self-
respecting nutritionist would call coffee a health food, one
cup in the morning, one and a half cups as a maximum, is
not likely to pose a measurable health hazard. The use of
caffeine has never been reliably linked to breast cancer, although some believe that it is associated with an increased
incidence of fibrocystic disorders of the breast. Many studies
do show that coffee consumption in excess of three cups daily
can contribute to increases in serum cholesterol levels and a
loss of calcium from the body. The only human cancer that
has been linked with caffeine and coffee use is pancreatic
cancer. A voluminous literature exists with both supporting
and negating results. When all of these studies are critically

considered, I believe there is no convincing evidence that coffee causes pancreatic cancer.

In a detailed description of the medical consequences of coffee use entitled "Wake Up and Smell the Coffee," Tony Chou, M.D., describes caffeine as the most widely consumed stimulant drug in the world, with about 75 percent ingested in the form of coffee.[162] More than half of all Americans drink coffee each day, with an average daily intake of two hundred milligrams of caffeine. (Of interest is the fact that coffee drinking is on the decrease in the United States. Higher amounts are consumed in Central and South America, and in Western Europe. The highest recorded consumption occurs in the United Kingdom and Scandinavia, where it is about double our intake. Also of interest is the fact that cigarette smoking accelerates caffeine metabolism; persons who stop smoking can have a doubling of the caffeine levels in the blood.)

Artificial sweeteners are not recommended as part of a health-supporting diet. They fall into the general category of chemicals, not food. Even though they have few calories, they do have sugarlike effects on serum insulin levels.

## About Alcohol

Is alcohol involved in the beginnings of breast cancer? After reviewing over two hundred scientific articles, I think it is fair to say that alcohol is an accepted risk factor, although not a strong one. This is confirmed in a number of international studies from Poland, Italy, France, Japan, England, Denmark, Australia, New Zealand, Norway, Russia, and the Netherlands.[163] They all support the observation that drinking alcohol, especially early in a woman's life, is associated with an increased incidence of breast cancer. The most dramatic risk increase was noted in Denmark, where re-

**Alcohol Risk Factor**

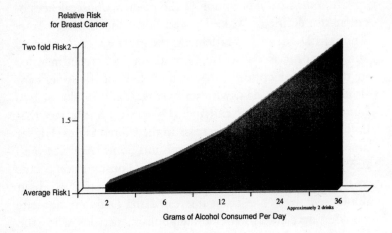

JAMA 260: 652-6, 1988

searchers found an eighteenfold increased risk among women drinking two drinks a day compared with nondrinkers.[164] However, other studies—including the excellent Framingham Heart Study—show no effect. One of the consistent findings in the positive studies was that the timing of the exposure to alcohol was important. Drinking during the early years was more harmful than drinking in later, adult years.

We also have studies informing us that alcohol suppresses our natural immunity. Some of this immunity is mediated by natural killer cells, whose activity is suppressed by alcohol.[165] Alcohol also suppresses white-blood-cell populations as well as being a source of free radicals. Alcohol alters the way that the liver metabolizes estrogen. Reichman and his associates at the National Institutes of Health in Bethesda, Maryland, found that two alcoholic beverages a day caused dramatic rises in estrone (21 percent), urinary estrone (15 percent), estradiol (22 percent), and estriol (29 per-cent).[166] Thus, the alcohol link to breast cancer seems solidly established. Prolonged increases in these hormone levels are a contributing factor to the development of breast cancer.

## About Milk

I recognize that milk and milk products are deeply rooted in both our culture and our cuisine. It is difficult to eliminate these products totally. I also recognize that many thousands of hardworking and self-reliant Americans work in the dairy industry. I am speaking strictly from the health standpoint as well as from the scientific standpoint as I view the evidence. After fully considering the dairy issue, I feel that optimal human health is best obtained without the use of even nonfat dairy products. Dairy products are also suspect in the development of another feared woman's disease, ovar-ian cancer. I realize that most nutritionists rely heavily on low-fat and nonfat dairy products. If you elect to use modest amounts of these products, it is true that the number of rec-ipes and dishes available to you is greatly increased. The one dairy product that I have a bit of scientific tolerance for is nonfat yogurt. This can be used in small amounts as a binder or as a vehicle for other foods and spices.

## About Meat and Cheese

"Men love meat and women love cheese"—this has been my observation after talking to hundreds of patients about their diets. Cheese is the second oldest manufactured food devised by humans; butter is the oldest. It is interesting that, in general, manufactured foods are not health-supporting.

Many people rely heavily on animal protein because they

were taught that it was the necessary center of a healthful diet. One of the great nutritional myths during the early and middle years of this century was: "You can't get enough good protein!" When I was young, any mention of the word *protein* was generally preceded by another word: *good*. A single five-ounce skinned chicken breast contains more than a day's allowance of protein for a 120-pound woman. Remember, too, that protein can be either of vegetable *or* animal origin. The animal variety comes with accompanying cholesterol, saturated fat, and sulfur-containing amino acids, while the vegetable variety comes with health-promoting fiber and complex carbohydrates. Incidentally, it is simply not true that complicated "combining schemes" are necessary to balance protein intake from vegetable and grain sources.[167] The average American woman eats much more than the recommended daily allowance of protein, occasionally even two or three times that amount. This not only contributes to obesity and cholesterol problems but also to osteoporosis. *Protein overload is a prime preventable cause of osteoporosis.* Cheese use should be limited to the very low-fat varieties, or none at all. Soy cheese, which also contains fat but no cholesterol, can be used in small amounts or grated on dishes for garnish and flavor. Low-fat and nonfat soy cheeses are now available. Meat use should be restricted to the RDA amounts for protein, preferably less, which allows the use of meat for garnish, flavor and accent, but not as the main portion of the meal.

## About Change

I've seen the puzzlement and concern that people have when confronting a new eating plan. I know because I went through it too. I can tell you this much: you must experience this food. You must try it. Many of us reject new ideas without a fair trial. It is not difficult to change; it is only difficult to start to change. It is also just as easy to make big changes instead of nibbling at the problem. If you are used to a typical American diet and you simply *think* about changing, you may feel overwhelmed. Your doctor is not likely to encourage you since physicians are often reluctant to recommend such eating plans and usually do not have the knowledge or understanding of truly modern nutrition to instruct you. Most doctors were not taught the benefits of a truly low-fat diet, do not know the benefits of a truly low-fat diet, don't eat properly themselves, and would not be comfortable imparting this type of information even if they possessed it.

If you make the suggested dietary changes and then "cheat" with an occasional fat-laden meal, you will be amazed at your body's reaction. You will feel stuffed, perhaps even have abdominal pains or cramps, and feel heavy and sluggish for hours. When you eat a fatty meal, the vital microcirculation of your body is sluggish and substantially impaired for up to twelve hours.

Your taste and food preferences will change when you switch to a reduced fat diet. A detailed article in the *American Journal of Clinical Nutrition*[168] found that after only three months on a low-fat diet, there was a lessening of pleasure associated with fatty and rich foods or beverages. This finding is in keeping with the common observations of persons who have converted to low-fat eating and who experience indigestion with the occasional high-fat meal.

Once you have embarked on a low-fat eating plan, you may find it difficult to persist without allies. Surround yourself with friends, associates, or family members who will aid and support you. Have a party where everyone brings a low-fat or nonfat dish. The last thing that you need is criticism or ribbing from unsympathetic, uninformed, or even envious persons. Avoid toxic people just as you would avoid toxic foods.

Let's keep our goals in mind and simply try to adapt to

them. If 20 percent fat intake is the minimum goal and 10 percent is the optimal goal, we can allow a small amount of fat, animal protein, or even dairy products, if desired, in the meal plan. As in so many other areas of life, the more effort you exert, the more you will gain. I find it difficult to count grams of fat each day; it just seems simpler to avoid as much fat as possible, remembering that even the plainest of foods usually contain 4 to 6-percent fat. The strategy presented here will put you into the 8 to 10-percent range. If you do decide to count grams of fat, an easy way to do so is to allow twenty-two grams of fat per day. This will represent less than 10 percent of calories if your total intake is two thousand calories per day. When fat *is* used, favor the monounsaturated and omega-3 types mentioned several times previously.

## Calculating Fat Content in Foods

To calculate the percentage of fat in a particular food, remember that each gram of fat contains nine calories. Next, read the label. For example, let's take a product that has one hundred calories per serving and contains three grams of fat. By multiplying the three fat grams by nine you get twenty-seven calories. You will obtain the percent of fat by dividing the fat calories by the total calories and shifting the decimal point two places to the right. This computes to 27 percent fat as calories. It's as simple as that. (The 27 is divided by 100, and the decimal is moved two places to the right.) I believe that the percent of calories from fat is the best way to compute fat intake. Your goal should be to keep this below 20 percent; 10 percent is even better.

Most Americans do not eat food from a great variety of recipes in a given week. According to one home economist, the average home cook has only ten main dishes in her repertoire for everyday meals. This doesn't include meals for festive or special occasions. People often eat the same thing, or very nearly the same thing, every day for breakfast; and some of my patients have had exactly the same breakfast each morning for years. Why? They say that they enjoy that particular breakfast and that it simplifies their morning routine. Another, larger group of people prefer to have the same meal, say, each Tuesday, or Friday night. If you can find just fifteen or twenty health-supporting meals that you truly enjoy and start rotating them, you will be nearly home free.

One way to make the transition from the traditional high-fat/low-fiber American diet to a cancer-prevention diet is to adopt some of our favorite ethnic dishes.

# 12

# Health-Supporting Food from Around the World

*A* health-supporting diet needn't be bland or boring. In fact, some of America's preferred ethnic cuisines—Italian, Chinese, Mexican, Thai, and Japanese—are easily incorporated into an eating plan for better health. After all, each of these countries has a lower breast cancer rate than the United States.

Let's start with *Italian* food and soups. The name *minestrone* seems automatically linked with Italian cuisine. Some of these soups are so substantial that they seem more like stews and would make a hearty meal when combined with a heavy, whole-grain bread. These soups often contain little or no meat. Minestrone is mixed with pasta or rice, and there are also traditional cabbage soups with carrots, celery, and beans. Lentil soups and pea soups are also popular. *Pasta e fagioli* (macaroni, beans, onions, carrots, tomatoes, garlic, olive oil, if desired, in small amounts, and seasoning—omit the ham, except perhaps for seasoning and flavor) is another traditional and health-supporting Italian soup.

Pasta is the mainstay of the evening meals in our home as it is in most of the homes in Italy. All eggless pastas are allowable. What is an acceptable pasta sauce? The most easily adapted is the marinara sauce based on tomato paste or fresh tomatoes, garlic, spices, and a greatly reduced amount of olive oil. Also delicious is a fresh pesto sauce made of pine nuts, basil, garlic, and olive oil. It will surprise some that pasta dishes can be very successful with only a small fraction of the usual amount of olive oil. Whole-wheat pastas (*pasta integrale*) are used widely in Italy as is whole-meal spaghetti (*bigoli*). Pasta primavera (pasta with steamed vegetables) with tomatoes, basil, garlic, and oregano is a wonderful and healthy main course. The list of health-supporting foods added to pasta is a long one. Garlic is the obligatory basic seasoning. Carrots, sweet peppers, hot pepper, zucchini, eggplant, cauliflower, mushrooms, onion, and tomatoes or tomato sauce are the other commonly used ingredients. Fish and shellfish in small quantities can be used if desired. Potato gnocchi (dumplings) with a tomato sauce is another favorite.

Risotto dishes using Italian short-grained rice (arborio) are wonderful and can be made without the usual large amounts of butter and oil. Defatted chicken broth or vegetable stock can be used. Any desired vegetable as well as the traditional mushrooms can be added. Lemon juice, wine, and spices add variety and flavor.

Polenta is a star, but watch for the butter and oil in many recipes. This staple, made from cornmeal, is commonly enjoyed in the north of Italy. Gnocchi, or small dumplings, mentioned above, can be made from cornmeal or mashed potatoes, which can be combined with vegetables such as spinach or garbanzo beans, or served with marinara sauce.

Pizza has an undeserved bad reputation. It can be healthful as well as delicious. The toppings can be any food that catches your fancy. Try peppers, tomatoes, onions, mushrooms, eggplant, and garlic. Be careful, though, about olive oil and cheese. It is not necessary to load a pizza with meat, cheese, and oil to have it taste great. Try it. Many pizza parlors will make an oilless pizza loaded with fresh vegetables, and just a little soy cheese, or no cheese at all.

Italian breads are varied and hearty and the vegetables are in enormous variety. Italian salads have introduced millions of Americans to radicchio, red chicory, and arugula. Mixed salad is fine provided you limit the olive oil. Enjoy balsamic vinegar instead. The same is true for spinach salad.

Italian desserts that are health-promoting include lemon sorbet and stuffed frozen oranges as well as the common fruit desserts. *Macedonia di frutta* is Italian fruit salad with a splash of optional orange liqueur. Even macaroons or *amaretti* made with egg whites are acceptable. *Granita* or fruit ice is a good hot-weather dish. Fruit (such as pears) poached in wine and spices are another favored Italian dessert. Major brand nonfat, non-cholesterol "Italian style" salad dressings are now widely available. They use guar gum, agar, and xanthan for "mouth feel" and thickening.

The great myth about American-style *Chinese* food is that it is health promoting. Unfortunately, it is laden with oil and protein, not to mention salt, sugar, and monosodium glutamate (MSG). How do we relate this to the good health reported in the recent Cornell-China Study? It seems that the American consumers of Chinese food have dictated to the providers of this food that it be "Americanized." Unfortunately, this has resulted in the addition of large amounts of meats and oils to the original cuisine. Do you know why the Chinese (in China) use such small amounts of oil and meats? Because it is scarce and expensive. There's simply not enough available for their huge populace. Recall their slimness and low cancer rates.

The secret to cooking stir-fried Chinese food healthily is to use a small amount of boiling water or vegetable stock not oil. It can be done! If you must use oil, use small amounts of peanut oil. Peanut oil is 31-percent linoleic acid, an essential fatty acid. Use either a standard wok or a Teflon-coated wok or pan. Here are two little-known methods to allow safer frying if you choose to use oils. Start by placing a small amount of water (vegetable stock is preferable if you have it) in the wok or pan. Then add your oil and ingredients, keeping the temperature in the moderate, not high ranges. The other method is to add the oil after the ingredients, again keeping the temperature down. Stir-fried vegetables, with tiny amounts of meat or shellfish for flavoring (optional) are simply wonderful. Ginger, soy sauce, garlic, and a drop or two of hot sesame or chili oil make the difference. However, steaming vegetables (or fish if desired) is preferable to frying, even low-fat stir-frying. Tofu is acceptable, especially when steamed, rather than fried. New, baked-flavor varieties of tofu are now available in many stores. Remember that tofu can be high in fat.

For our purposes, Chinese soups are based on a vegetable stock made from chopped vegetables, garlic, ginger, pepper, and coriander. Bean curd (tofu), cellophane noodles, and vegetable soups are easy to prepare and are delicious. Water chestnuts, Chinese cabbage or bok choy, bamboo shoots, snow peas, and a variety of noodles are just a few of the wonderful ingredients available in what many experts feel is the most varied cuisine on this earth. Hot-and-sour soup fits our guidelines and wonton soup is also fine if the usual large amounts of pork are omitted. Vegetable wonton is excellent. Broth soups with vegetables, noodles, and meat or seafood for flavoring are acceptable. Defatted chicken broth is available in most stores.

Rice is, of course, the basic Chinese food. We are most familiar with steamed, white rice. Try brown rice. It is often used in China, tastes great, and is preferable nutritionally to white rice. In much of the Orient, rice is eaten at all meals, even for breakfast. (On a recent visit to China, I was told that the Chinese consume more millet than rice, but that they prefer the rice.) Basmati rice smells and tastes particularly good, even if it originates in India rather than China.

Desserts are not an emphasized part of Chinese cookery, but litchi nuts, kumquats, and perhaps a nonfat lime sorbet would fit well.

*Mexican* food is a natural for our dietary plan. Corn tortillas, beans, rice, and salsa are the mainstays. Even flour tortillas are now available in a fat-free version. Whole-wheat nonfat tortillas have been available for some time. Warmed tortillas can be filled with a variety of foods. Tamales, enchiladas, tacos, tostadas, and burritos can all be prepared to our guidelines and are delicious. Salsa provides flavor and color, without fat, and with minimal calories. You can easily prepare your own with chopped onions, tomatoes, peppers, garlic, and cilantro.

Black-bean soup and gazpacho are excellent choices. Black-bean fillings or nonfat refried bean fillings (in the place of meats) are delicious and easy to prepare. The main trick here is not to get a large amount of lard in the refried beans, or oil in the tortillas. Nonfat refried canned beans are now available in most well-stocked supermarkets. Watch the labels for these ingredients. Another problem spot in the traditional Mexican diet is an emphasis on cheese. Many dishes are just as appealing with little or no cheese.

*Japanese* food is naturally low in fat, as we've mentioned before. But be aware that the Japanese themselves have steadily increased the fat in their diet as they have succumbed to Western ways. Miso soups meet our guidelines, but are high in salt. The traditional Japanese cucumber salad is excellent. Steamed rice or cooked noodles with steamed vegetables is ideal for our plan. Sukiyaki and sushi are fine, but avoid raw fish or tempura, which is deep-fried and very high in fat.

*Indian* food has an ancient tradition of vegetarianism. Mulligatawny soup or *dal* (lentil soup) are standards. The Indian breads are nothing less than fabulous. *Chapatis* and *roti* are fine, but watch for the *naan* or *poori*, which have more fat. Basmati rice, *pappadams*, and pilaf are standards. The variety, complexity, and fragrance of the spices are wondrous. I spent a year in Ceylon and several months in India, and the vegetarian food I enjoyed there is still a vivid memory. Watch out for *ghee* (clarified butter) and milk products, though.

*French* food has been long associated with the finest in the world's gourmet eating. Can this cuisine be reconciled with our guidelines? After all, when we think of this food, we automatically think of butter, eggs, cream, rich cheeses, cream sauces, and beef. Despite all this, the answer is yes. French food can be adapted to our requirements. The older classical French cuisine is heavier and richer—and therefore more dangerous—than the newer and lighter *nouvelle cuisine*. Onion soup without the cheese topping can serve as a starter along with French bread. The French vegetable soups, often tomato-based, are excellent. Consommés are also fine. Salads are certainly a mainstay with the French insistence on freshness of ingredients. Salad niçoise is fine with small amounts of water-packed tuna and without the egg yolk and oil. Appetizers are excellent in the French cuisine. Crudités (selected, sliced raw vegetables) are a standard. Steamed and baked vegetables are also a standby. Entrées are safest when steamed or poached, occasionally baked. Ratatouille (baked eggplant, zucchini, and tomatoes) is a delicious vegetable casserole. When dining in French restaurants, ask if your entrée can be prepared without butter or oil. For dessert, the usual fresh fruit and wonderful poached pears or other seasonal fruits are *magnifique*.

*Greek* food fits fairly well within our plan. The major problem is to enlist some restraint with the added olive oil. Despite the fact that olive oil is probably the least dangerous of all the oils, it still is not recommended as a health food. Greek salads are delicious and varied. Tomato salad alone, cucumber salad, carrot-and-cabbage salad, cabbage-and-tomato salad are standards. The dressings tend to combine olive oil, vinegar, lemon juice, mint, and chopped olives. Soups include potato, lentil, chickpea, bean, vegetable, and rice with lemon. Pasta is alive and well in Greece. *Pastitsio* is a classically Greek dish. Watch the butter and cheese, though. Artichokes are used in a variety of dishes. *Dolmades*, or stuffed grape leaves, are perfect if the olive oil is not too heavy and meat is omitted. *Moussaka* (potato, eggplant, zucchini casserole) can be prepared in a number of ways with or without meat and olive oil. Another standard is spinach pie (*spanakopita*). Milk and butter must be eliminated to meet our needs. Stuffed tomatoes can work for us, while grilled, mixed vegetables are perfect—just hold the butter. The Greeks enjoy a variety of stews that can be readily adapted to our guidelines.

## Other Cuisines

*Thai* cooking is wondrous and has many marvelous dishes with exotic names, flavors, and aromas. From the *Middle East* comes *tabbouli*, a bulgur-wheat salad including parsley, onion, and tomatoes that can be prepared to our guidelines. Vegetable or curry couscous from North Africa is an interesting entrée that will work well for added variety.

*German* sauerkraut, potatoes, and some very fine non-oil breads are about all that can be salvaged from that cuisine, which has the highest fat percentage recently recorded, 49 percent of calories. In keeping with the theme of this book, since shortly after World War II, German women have developed a high rate of breast cancer. Even their men have extremely high rates of breast cancer.

There are foods that are acceptable for us from every cuisine on record. After all, peasant food was the dominant food of every culture, and peasant food is almost always health-supporting food. Look for the old, traditional, and simple dishes that sustained humans for thousands of years. It's as simple as that.

Some of our experts claim that a breast-cancer-prevention diet is "culturally unacceptable" and is "socially isolating." I think those phrases are at the same time insulting and patronizing. *It is breast cancer that is unacceptable.*

While it is relatively easy to find and prepare health-supporting foods in your own kitchen, dining out can sometimes pose a challenge. How can you enjoy restaurant fare and still follow the plan set forth in this book? It's not as hard as you might think.

# 13

# The Kradjian Guide to Restaurant Eating

More than 40 percent of the American individual food budget is spent eating out according to an article in—of all places—the *Journal of the American Medical Association* of December 19, 1990. This article states that the number of dining establishments is expected to increase by 30 percent over the next decade. Another survey tells us that the average American eats out about 190 times a year.

When you either choose to, or must, eat in a restaurant, you are in the enemy's camp. But all is not lost. Following is the Kradjian guide to restaurant eating—strategies and techniques that will help you when you venture into "hostile" territory.

Whenever possible, patronize only restaurants that offer healthful choices. The fine people who operate today's restaurants are dedicated professionals to be sure, but their main reason for opening their doors each day is an economic one. If they realize that the public will not continue to eat the food that has contributed to the early death of so many, they *will* change their offerings. It is our duty to help them do so.

The future of our food supply is in the hands of the consumer, not the food industry, the government, or an advertising agency. *We* are in control, and without our dollars, nothing happens. If there are no restaurants offering health-supporting food, clearly inform the owners that unless such choices are made available, they will lose your patronage.

Let's imagine a typical situation. You are traveling cross-country by car and simply must eat in an average American restaurant. What to do? The challenge is to learn how to choose.

Start by studying the menu. Then order a salad. Usually there will be a garden salad or a mixed green salad or a dinner salad, all representing inoffensive, if also unexciting, lettuce, tomatoes, sprouts, etc. The real problem is with the dressing. You are usually asked, "What dressing would you like?" An expected response would be thousand island, or ranch, or blue cheese. Instead, ask for oil and vinegar on the side. When this arrives, use the vinegar and ignore the oil, or use only a small amount. (With *any* salad dressing, ask for the dressing on the side so that you control the amount used.) A wedge of lemon is another possibility for a salad dressing. Ask for a dinner roll or whole-wheat bread and don't use the usual packaged soda crackers. Ignore the butter. You might ask if they happen to have a nonfat, noncholesterol salad dressing. Do not settle for the usual "low-cal" dressings, which are anything but low in calories and fat. Watch for salad dressings that claim to be fat-free but are not. Check the list of ingredients.

The next item is soup. Often there will be one or more soups that are perfectly acceptable just as they appear on the menu. On other occasions you will have to ask for the soup of the day. What you are looking for is a non-cholesterol, nonfat soup, or as close to that as possible. Vegetable soup is a natural; minestrone is about the same. Bean soup, lentil soup, split-pea soup, borsht, and many noodle soups are all acceptable. If they are cooked with beef, chicken, or turkey, you can make a decision. Either remove the meat and enjoy the residual flavoring, remove a portion of the meat, or just eat the soup as is. One category of soups to avoid altogether when dining out is cream soups. Pastina and broth soups are fine. Mushroom, tomato, and corn soups are good if there is no added milk or cream.

Occasionally there will be a main dish that you can eat as is. It is highly unlikely that this will be a standard American dish, since our cuisine is so deeply rooted in the meat-centered, high-fat tradition. Even with a vegetarian entrée, the nearly obligatory addition of oils, butter, cream, and cheese usually makes these plates unacceptable. The ethnic possibilities one might find in an average American restaurant would include spaghetti with marinara sauce or pasta primavera. Always ask for the sauce to be served on the side. This gives you the control over the amount used. On rare occasions, you may find some Mexican entrées such as bean tacos, enchiladas, or tostadas, which are acceptable if lard is not included in the bean mix. Ask them to prepare the dish with no cheese. Also, ask that the tortillas be steamed and not fried. In the average neighborhood restaurant, pasta is probably the safest choice, another is the baked potato.

Another standby is the good old American sandwich. The bread for the sandwich should be whole wheat, though pita, rye, or French breads are also acceptable. (You do give up fiber with the French-bread choice.) For the filling, you have two choices: either order the "least dangerous" and simply eat it as is, or remove some of the meat. An example would be a turkey sandwich with lettuce, tomato, and onions, but without mayonnaise. You can leave a small amount of turkey for the flavor. The other course is to ask the waitress or waiter to custom-make a sandwich to your specifications. Of course, "Hold the mayo" should be your invariable request unless they have one of the new nonfat, noncholesterol varieties. Mustard is acceptable.

Don't forget the good old baked potato. This is a wonderful standby as long as the topping is served on the side to give you control. Cooked beans are a perfect topping. Chives and chopped broccoli, barbecue sauce, and salsa are also fine. Potatoes are delicious just by themselves with a little black pepper and salt.

Tell the waiter—directly and simply—what you require. Be clear, pleasant, and definite. This may solve all of your restaurant problems. Certainly, if you plan to eat at the same restaurant for a number of meals, this makes the most sense. Don't forget to tip properly when you get special attention.

One more tactic is to order double portions of desired and safe foods, such as vegetables, potatoes, etc., and skip the customary meat-based entrée.

We have been talking about an average American restaurant, but the choices are much wider if you find a buffet. Here you should have no trouble whatever in meeting your requirements. The problem might instead lie in the temptation to cheat just a little with all that "free" food beckoning to you. At least one national chain of buffet restaurants, Fresh Choice, offers a variety of clearly marked nonfat and noncholesterol food choices.

The demand for well-prepared, delicious, and health-supporting food may become so great that many, or even most, of the restaurants in your area will offer this type of fare. This is the case in the Santa Rosa area (Northern California) chiefly due to the efforts of one of my medical colleagues, Dr. John McDougall, whose radio programs and writings have sparked a true diner rebellion in that community. Because of their insistence on delicious food that is also health-supporting, there are now over seventy restaurants that offer as part of their menu exactly the oilless, dairyless, and meatless food that we have been discussing. I've had the pleasure of dining in that area a half-dozen times, and it's wonderful. Encourage the restaurant owners in your area to make changes. Eventually economic realities alone will foster this trend. Never underestimate the power of the American dollar or the American entrepreneurial spirit.

Two recent polls of restaurant owners indicate an increasing willingness to accommodate the health-conscious diner. Nearly 70 percent of restaurateurs surveyed by MasterCard said that asking for a menu switch was not a problem. The National Restaurant Association said that 90 percent of their members would be willing to serve a sauce or salad dressings on the side, and that 80 percent would broil or bake an item rather than fry it on request.[169]

You now know the basic principles of the Kradjian plan, as well as how to maintain your program of dietary change even while dining out. You are ready to take those steps that I firmly believe will help save yourself from breast cancer. "But, Dr. Kradjian," you may ask, "what if you're wrong?"

# 14

## *What If I'm Wrong?*

*T*his is an important chapter, even though it is a short one. What if the link between dietary fat, dietary fiber, and breast cancer were nonexistent? In other words, what if everything I have been telling you about breast cancer and diet is false, is absolutely incorrect? What would be the health consequences of adopting the diet plan described here? In short, *what if I am altogether wrong?*

Even if that were the case—and I don't believe for a moment that it is—a woman following this plan would be greatly protected against a long list of other diseases. Not to mention that your risk of developing breast cancer would be completely unchanged! That would leave you with a one-out-of-eight lifetime risk of developing breast cancer. But wait, that leaves you with a seven-out-of-eight chance that you will not have breast cancer. If you are not exposed to breast cancer, then you will be exposed to a one-in-two probability of developing heart disease, a one-in-three chance of diabetes, and one-in-five possibility of a stroke, or a one-in-seven risk of hip fracture.

Following the plan we advocate will protect you, at least partially, against all these disorders. How is this possible? It is possible only because an eating plan such as I am advocating provides the exact substances, the precise fuel, required by our bodies for good health. There is ample, well-documented, scientific support that this diet provides substantial protection against heart disease, diabetes, stroke, and hip fracture. Why? It is the diet that the human body was designed for. By contrast, the standard American high-fat/low-fiber diet is a recipe for the following familiar disasters, and there is a long list of other diseases and disorders that could be added:

- heart disease
- cancer
- stroke
- diabetes
- obesity
- gallstones
- diverticulitis
- arthritis
- for men, prostate cancer

Some of these diseases are lethal; others such as diverticulitis are quite serious, and even others are merely painful. We've had a hundred years to consider this. We are not "adapting" to our improper diet; instead we are suffering and dying from it. So, even if I am wrong about the breast-cancer-prevention part of my diet, following this eating plan will be a great aid to your overall health and the health of your family and friends. What greater legacy can you leave your children than to teach them to live healthily?

Although this is a book about breast cancer, prostate cancer must be mentioned. The American Cancer Society predicts 200,000 new patients with prostate cancer in 1994 in the United States, some 20,000 more than will diagnosed with breast cancer. Most American women live with, or at least are vitally concerned about the health of one or more men. Prostate cancer has virtually identical risk factors to the breast cancer risk factors listed in this book. This allows a married couple, for example, to enthusiastically embark together on this breast and prostate cancer reduction plan.

But there's another side to this question. What if I'm right? What if everything said about the prevention of breast cancer is correct? What will be the result if thousands, or hundreds of thousands, of women take up the challenge and reduce their fat intake to truly protective levels, increase their dietary fiber, increase the amounts of antioxidants eaten, and implement an exercise program? Here is where things become a bit vague. To all intents and purposes, nothing will happen. *There will be no victims.* There will be no apparent effect. The only thing that will eventually become evident is that the statisticians will start speaking of a "new trend" or a "leveling off" of breast cancer, which they will assert had already started in the early 1990s. In any event, fewer women will become breast cancer victims, but which ones were spared? Who was saved?

This is the *paradox of prevention.* When you have a cancer to treat, people are remarkably focused in their efforts to defeat that tumor. Even if the therapy is botched, or ineffective, even harsh or crude, the patients and their families are often profoundly—even inappropriately—grateful. Insurance companies are also appreciative, and issue generous checks to the medical providers. Pharmaceutical companies prosper, hospitals are busy, accountants, administrators, vendors, medical-supply people—all are profitably occupied.

By contrast *when someone is spared from breast cancer by preventative measures, we won't even know who it was!* There is not only no personal recognition for medical professionals; there is no glory, no credit, no awards, and no profit. It seems as if it just didn't happen. That's what prevention is, something that didn't happen. And that is why prevention is an orphan—there's no obvious payoff, just lives saved. How can we count those lives? Some will say that maybe lives were saved, but the trend was headed downward anyway. Others think that I'm underestimating the ability of our statisticians, and that they should be able to correlate fat disappearance data plotted against breast cancer rates. Do you think our society and our institutions are mature enough to tolerate prevention? It certainly won't be good for business!

When this situation is analyzed using game-theory techniques, there are only four possibilities. Both of the possible outcomes are beneficial if our advice is followed. By contrast, if our advice is ignored, the possibilities are either very dangerous or there will be no change.

### GAME THEORY ANALYSIS

|  | ADVICE FOLLOWED | ADVICE IGNORED |
|---|---|---|
| If We're **Right** | Significant reduction in breast cancer risk as well as heart disease, stroke, diabetes, etc. | Disaster |
| If We're **Wrong** | No reduction in breast cancer risk, but great reduction in heart disease, stroke, etc. | Neutral. Nothing gained, nothing lost. |

It is apparent that there is *nothing to lose* by adopting the advice offered in this book. And if the advice is correct (which I fully believe it to be), ignoring the advice would be disastrous.

If you want to avoid breast cancer, learn to live like the billions of women on this planet who are already avoiding this dread disease! Never give up the battle to stay fit and live well. Good health to you! You deserve it!

# 15

# *For Doctors Only*

T he rest of you can relax and ignore this section; it is for my fellow physicians. All right, doctors, I know, I know! You're finding all this tough to swallow. You just can't believe that all the things you were taught about breast cancer in medical school and thereafter are a little off-line, just a bit out of focus.

## A Friendly Challenge

Here is my challenge to you if you are still skeptical about the association between diet, lifestyle, and breast cancer.

Show me any large group of women—anywhere on earth—who are reliably known to be following a long-term, low-fat diet, who also have a high incidence of breast cancer. That is part one of the challenge.

Here's part two—please show me a group of women—anywhere on earth—who chronically eat a high-fat diet and who also have a low incidence of breast cancer.

I know that in any group of persons studied for any

biological phenomenon, there will be the odd case, the exception, the outlier. Let's not waste our time on oddities, peripheral issues, and individuals at the ends of the normal distribution curve. Let's concentrate on the main, central, and dominant tendencies of these groups.

I would define a low-fat diet for the purposes of this challenge as a diet with total calories from fat at *15 percent or less*. Please don't quibble and say, "No one lives on that low a fat intake." There are many more women on earth who live on such a low-fat diet than who live on our Western high-fat diet! A high-fat diet, for the purpose of our challenge, is 35 to 40 percent of total calories from fat. This is not a farfetched value. In the Harvard Nurses' Study, many of the women admitted to "49 percent or more of energy from fat"; that would probably make their actual values closer to 55 percent.

I feel the challenge has already been met. *This work has been done.* For years, investigators have combed the files of tumor registries and hospital records all over the world looking for these associations, and the results have been published. As if it were an immutable law of life or nature—as indeed it is—those populations of women with low-fat diets have low breast cancer rates. Those populations of women with high-fat diets have high rates of breast cancer. *There are no exceptions.* Do not be misled by studies that focus only on high-risk women and omit a low-fat study group. The best-known example of this type of investigation is the Harvard Nurses' Study.

If that were not enough to convince a fair-minded person, it must be noted that there are over a dozen reliable migration studies that clearly show increases in breast cancer when women simply move from a low-cancer-incidence country to a high-cancer-incidence country—but only if they adopt the diet and lifestyle of the new country. If they remain in an ethnic enclave while in the new country and do not change their diet, there is little or no increase in their breast cancer rate. These studies have been nicely documented, particularly among Asian women migrating to Hawaii.

When an impartial observer analyzes the data on breast cancer and diet as seen around the world, another fact is noted: increased dietary fat is associated particularly with increased *postmenopausal* breast cancer rates. This fits with the data previously presented for the following reasons: any true genetic factor is more likely to express itself early in life rather than late. Environmental factors, on the other hand, are cumulative and are thus time- and dose-related; that is, the longer the suspected factors are in play, the greater the effect, and those effects would be more likely to be postmenopausal.

Another fascinating aspect of the dietary fat issue derives from an analysis of the proportion of fat from animal or vegetable sources. There is a consistent and high correlation between consumption of animal fat and animal protein, and breast cancer. There is a weak correlation between vegetable fat and breast cancer. This is somewhat surprising when one reviews the animal experiments that clearly show increasing breast cancer rates with increasing vegetable oil intakes. It may be that the degree of saturation of the vegetable oil and the relative lack of risk compared to animal-fat sources are the keys. In any event, the data are clear. Cereal, whole grains, vegetable, and fruit intake is protective against breast cancer. Meat, milk, butter, oil, and egg intake is conducive to high breast cancer rates.

As mentioned, the same data apply to prostate cancer, with a strong positive correlation with calories of animal origin and a negative one with vegetable-derived calories. Carcinoma of the ovary also is strikingly similar to breast cancer in many of the respects discussed above. Cancer of the colon also can be correlated to per capita fat consumption.

When discussing a low-fat eating plan and breast cancer

prevention, a logical and important question is: "How low is low enough?" or "What level of fat intake is protective?" There are very few scientific studies that specifically address this important question. One of these comes from P. G. Toniolo at the famous Cancer Institute in Milan. In a 1989 study[170] he found a reduced risk for breast cancer only when total calories derived from fat was less than 28 percent. A similar reduction was found for less than 10 percent of calories as saturated fat or less than 6 percent of calories as animal proteins. This study was of further interest as it indicates that these reduced levels of fat and protein are protective in adult life. He had earlier reported that the reduction in fat was particularly critical in the years surrounding puberty.

Leonard Cohen, David Rose, and Ernst Wynder are pioneers in scientific nutritional study. After an extensive review of epidemiological studies, animal experiments, and feasibility studies, they suggest a dietary goal of 15 percent of total calories as fat for the prevention of breast cancer.[171]

The 28-percent-fat figure cited by Toniolo is probably the most lenient to be found in the scientific literature as possibly conferring protection against breast cancer. If there is a drawback in the breast-cancer-prevention plan presented in this book, it is that the changes necessary to prevent cancer are not small, extremely easy to make, or simply cosmetic. Cutting down on red meat and eating plenty of chicken and fish *is just not enough*. We are advocating substantial changes, not just a "wave" in the direction of a reduced fat diet. Remember the key work of Dr. T. Colin Campbell, who learned that the lowest rates of breast cancer in China were found in areas where the women ate 6 percent of their calories as fat. There is *no known lower limit* to the protective threshold for an excellent diet. The more you do, the more you'll gain. Remember that the "worst" women in the China study ate only 24 percent of their calories as fat; and they had higher levels of breast cancer than their sisters who consumed the very lowest levels.

Remember where the fat comes from in our diet. The United States Department of Agriculture says that:

| | |
|---|---|
| Meat, poultry, and fish provide | 44 percent of our daily fat |
| Dairy foods provide | 13 percent of our daily fat |
| Oils and visible fat provide | 11 percent of our daily fat |
| Grains provide | 14 percent of our daily fat |
| *All other* sources provide | <u>18</u> percent of our daily fat |
| | 100 percent |

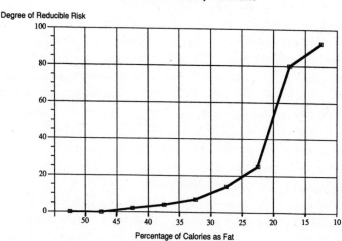

**Reduction of Breast Cancer Risk
As Related to Dietary Fat Intake**

With over two thirds of our fat intake from meat, dairy products and oils, it is easy to know where to start trimming.

At the end of the debate, there is really only one crucial question: "Is breast cancer chiefly an environmental disease?" If it is, our currently agreed-upon medical approach is *essentially incorrect*. We have been in error many times before in the history of medicine. A few examples include the case of 100 percent oxygen for premature infants, the treatment of diverticulitis before Dr. Denis Burkitt, the Sippy Diet for peptic ulcers, and high-fat diets for diabetics.

I firmly believe that the totality of the evidence does support the conclusion that breast cancer is chiefly an environmental disease. And if environmental, it is chiefly dietary, and therefore it is chiefly preventable. Carefully consider all the evidence without preconceptions and make your own conclusions; your patients, your families, and you yourself deserve the best.

# ∽ 16

## *What I've Learned*

Why have I been troubling American women with the sometimes distressing information contained in this volume? Why am I inconveniencing you? It is because there is a marvelous opportunity to be seized. That opportunity is the potential extension of vigorous, effective human life. My thesis is that for many American women, premature deaths can be avoided. A corollary to this belief is that we are born healthy, but make ourselves ill with our personal choices and lifestyle. The lifestyle choices discussed in this book, if acted upon, will improve health and extend effective and useful years—perhaps by a great number.

What to do with that time is the *real* essence of living. This is an intensely personal matter. Each woman has her own vision. No doctor may properly intrude upon it. To many, it is watching and participating in the lives of their children and their grandchildren; or perhaps even great-grandchildren. I find this to be the most mentioned goal set aside for the "bonus years" women hope to gain. Younger women are looking forward to raising their children and nurturing their family or their career. Others have more specific or material goals. A trip around the world or to Europe is often mentioned, or perhaps a leisurely tour around our own great country. Involvement in absorbing hobbies—reading, painting, and music have been mentioned. To be involved with pleasure-oriented groups or more serious service organizations is another common goal. For a good many, their religious activities are paramount. This is for you to decide. Our task is to help you to achieve the goal—a long, healthy life.

I hope that this book gives you some of the knowledge to achieve the goal. If you can later share the knowledge with those you love, and they in turn benefit, that would be the crowning achievement.

If you want to avoid breast cancer, then learn to live like the billions of women on this earth who will avoid this disease. Women in the protected countries eat less than 20 to 40 grams of fat each day. In the countries with high breast cancer rates, the women ingest over 100 grams of fat daily. *Eat as the women in protected countries do*—a diet high in protective vegetables, fruits, and fiber, a plant-based diet. Stress the complex carbohydrates, avoid the simple sugars. Avoid alcohol. Avoid pesticides. Avoid excessive protein loads, especially proteins from animal sources. Become lean and stay lean. Become and stay physically active. Protect yourself at all times and never give up in the battle for good health. Learning to live well is a continuing process.

## ∞ *Appendix 1*

## *Harvard and the Harvard Nurses' Study*

*I*n the early 1980s and the early 1990s, information on dietary fat and breast cancer was beginning to make an impact on the thinking of American women. A flood of magazine articles became the main conduit for this information.

And then something happened. It was the publication of a single article in the *Journal of the American Medical Association* of October 21, 1992. The article was entitled "Dietary Fat and Fiber in Relation to Risk of Breast Cancer: An 8-Year Follow-up," also called the "Harvard Nurses' Health Study." Eight of the nine authors of this study, headed by Walter C. Willett, M.D., were based at the Harvard Department of Nutrition.

Radio, television, and newspaper reports of this study swept the land, telling us that there was "no connection between dietary fat and breast cancer."

Here is how the press reported it in a headline from the *San Francisco Chronicle*: STUDY FINDS NO LINK BETWEEN DIET AND BREAST CANCER RISK. One expert was quoted as saying, "This is an excellent study," and, "If your goal is to do something really substantial about breast cancer risk, you're wasting your time with fat reduction." From the October 21, 1992, *Los Angeles Times*: STUDY FINDS NO LINK OF FAT IN DIET TO MALIGNANCY RISK. A newscaster said, "So go ahead, order that cheeseburger." The United Press International reported, BREAST CANCER RISK UNAFFECTED BY FAT CONSUMPTION, October 20, 1992. On the same date, Reuters Limited put it this way, STUDY FINDS NO FAT OR FIBER LINK TO BREAST CANCER. The Associated Press offered, LOW-FAT, HIGH-FIBER DIET NO PROTECTION AGAINST BREAST CANCER, STUDY SAYS.

The Harvard Nurses' Health Study began in 1976, when 121,701 nurses (all women) who lived in eleven states returned mailed questionnaires concerning their medical histories and lifestyle. By 1992, the study involved 89,494 of these same nurses, aged thirty-four through fifty-nine years, who had been followed up for eight years.

Why am I taking time here to tell you of this study? It is simply because this particular scientific study has become identified as a definitive work, the last word, on the subject of breast cancer and dietary fat. Not only has a deep impression been made on the thinking of the public and the media, but most of the doctors in America also seem willing to accept its conclusions. I feel that those conclusions are disastrously wrong.

After looking at this study in considerable detail, you can make up your own mind as to whether the authors' conclusions are justified. You can decide whether the Harvard doctors are giving you true and reliable information. You decide whether you can rely on the editors of the *Journal of the American Medical Association* to always choose articles with valid conclusions. You do not have to be a scientist to make these decisions. Your good sense and good judgment will be more than sufficient.

The Harvard Nurses' Health Study is a cohort study. This simply means that there is no study group and no con-

**Harvard Nurses' Study**

Percentage of
Calories as Fat

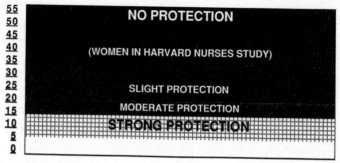

Source: Chart R.M. Kradjian, M.D. 1994

trol group. An entire group of women was studied, and associations—or the lack of them—were sought between a disease (in this case, breast cancer) and other factors (for example, fat and fiber). One prominent researcher, Dr. Ernst Wynder, says that this type of study "is the weakest link in the chain of evidence relating to the dietary fat hypothesis." For example, if all, or nearly all, women in a group follow dangerous health practices, there will be little or no difference in the risk of the disease between the "best" and the "worst" of such a group.

Consider this comparative example. If you wish to learn the effect of speed on automobile safety, you might measure motor-vehicular deaths in a group of motorists driving 90 to 120 miles per hour. If you did this, you would find little difference in death rates among the 90- or 95-mile-per-hour drivers compared with the 110- or 115-mile-per-hour motorists. A "logical" conclusion could then be made that "speed has nothing whatever to do with motor-vehicular fatalities," which is, of course an erroneous statement. That is essentially what the Harvard study has done! By following a group of women ingesting from 27 to over 50 percent of calories as fat (average 39 percent in their 1980 group and 33 percent in their 1984 group), they were looking at a group all of whom were at risk to develop breast cancer. After all, these are American women, and that is precisely the group of women that we are so concerned about. And it is American women, this very group, that have been experiencing the rise in breast cancer rates that we have been lamenting. Therefore, these women were all at risk because of their high-fat diet, and that is what the study confirmed.

Further, the Harvard Nurses' Health Study was nothing more than a giant mail survey. I verified this by talking to over forty of the nurses who were subjects of the study. Not one of them saw or even talked to the Harvard researchers. This was more like a poll than a scientific study in the ordinarily accepted sense of the word.

In the mailed questionnaire, the nurses were asked to recall on average how often and in what amount they consumed a variety of foods over the preceding two years. There were nine possible responses, ranging from *never* to *six or more times per day.* Just think of the problem you would have in recalling what you ate over the past two years!

One nurse I spoke with confirmed that there was never any personal or telephone contact with the researchers. She was conscientious in filling out the questionnaires, which she described as a "nightmare." She found it impossible to recall not only the details, but even the broad outlines, of her dietary intake over the preceding two years. She recalled being troubled that there were seasonal patterns to her food intake and no way to reflect this accurately in the questionnaire. She also became more aware of the importance of nutrition during the course of the study and radically changed her diet. During the study, several of her family members developed breast cancer. There was no provision for reporting this, and she found herself writing the changes along the margins of her questionnaire. When asked if she thought she may have indulged some unconscious "fudging" downward of her estimates of fat intake, she answered that she may have.

During the eight years of the follow-up in the Harvard study, 1.7 percent of the original study group died, and 1,566 cases of breast cancer were recorded. Of these cases, 127 were described as in situ (or noninvasive) lesions and were discarded. Why? These are the earliest cancer lesions in the breast and make up a very significant portion of our breast cancer patients at present—28 percent of all new breast cancer patients at one of our local hospitals.[172] Why did the Harvard study show only 8 percent? In addition, eighty cases of breast cancer were included in which there was no pathology report! A serious discussion of breast cancer without an absolute microscopic tissue confirmation is a first in my thirty-five years of reading medical journals. What was accepted in those eighty cases, the word of someone's relative in a telephone call or letter? This would not even amount to responsible newspaper work, let alone high-level scientific investigation.

Next, the women were arranged into arbitrary quintiles or fifths, based on their responses to the questionnaires. That is, the women were divided into five equal groups that were then considered "low" to "high" for the studied variable. These quintiles were then compared with regard to a number of variable factors, some of which are listed below. The most important of these variables was, of course, dietary fat. This was broken down into categories: saturated fat, unsaturated fat, monounsaturated fat, and cholesterol. The study's reported findings were often contrary to proven effects of fat and other foods on health.

Here is a listing of some of the questionable findings from the Harvard Nurses' Health Study. When the lowest usage group for fat was compared with the highest usage group, there were reported to be *fewer* cancer cases in the group that consumed the most fat. The Harvard scientists inform us that the group eating the *most* fat had fewer breast cancer cases than the group who ate the *least* fat. It would appear that fat is protective against breast cancer if we can believe these figures. (Remember that there are hundreds of scientific papers that tell us just the opposite.)

They also report that increasing the amount of dietary fiber offered no protection whatever. Even an increased intake of cholesterol seemed to have a beneficial effect in reducing breast cancer levels, but only if the woman was postmenopausal.

One finding claimed that increasing the total fat intake for the 89,000 plus women was associated with increased slimness and smallness! The highest fat-intake group was smaller and lighter than the lowest fat-intake group. Does this fit with the reality that you have experienced and observed during your lifetime? This study design tells us that high cholesterol protects against breast cancer, and fat makes you thinner!

The next section is so bizarre that I feel in fairness I must accurately and fully quote from the *Journal of the American Medical Association* study: "Apart from alcoholic beverages, which were positively related to risk, the only other significant association was an inverse relation with cake." And: "We observed nonsignificant inverse trends with consumption of meats and desserts." (An inverse relation or trend confers protection.) The Harvard scientists did not specify whether the cake was layer cake, chocolate cake, or other.

In other words, in a hugely expensive, highly regarded, eight-year, continuing study of over 89,000 women, only two solid, statistically significant findings emerged. Here they are again, brace yourself! Alcohol is a risk factor and cake protects! One might conclude that if you want to protect yourself from breast cancer, avoid alcohol and eat a lot of cake! Marie Antoinette said it first. Believe it or not, I did find one additional reference to cake in my perusal of the scientific literature on breast cancer. A Japanese study found that a large intake of cake produced an *increased* risk of breast cancer of nearly twofold (relative risk = 1.83).[173]

There are even more amazing conclusions. From a chart in the study, one can learn that increasing your fat intake to 47 percent of total calories will afford you a 20-percent lessened rate of breast cancer compared with women ingesting less than 29 percent of calories as fat. Fat does not protect you from breast cancer. To me, this reveals a flawed study design as there are at least eleven other similar studies that have contrary findings.

Even beef fat may be helpful in reducing breast cancer risk, according to the Harvard researchers! After noting that monounsaturated fat was protective, the authors observe that "the largest source of monounsaturated fat intake in our study population was beef fat. Further examination of the relationship between monounsaturated fat intake and breast cancer risk is clearly warranted." Is this paper sponsored by the Beef Board? Does anyone believe that the way to reduce breast cancer is to eat fatty cuts of beef?

In the fine print at the end of the nine-page article is an insignificant-looking notice advising the reader that twelve pages of "supplementary material" is available for $7.75. This is NAPS document No. 04978 and can be obtained from Microfiche Publications, P.O. Box 3513, Grand Central Station, New York, New York, 10163–3513. If you are truly interested in the details of the Harvard Nurses' Study, you must read this material. If you do, you will find some surprises.

Do you like ice cream? According to the supplemental data available by mail, ice cream weakly protects against breast cancer. The more whole milk, yogurt, and cheese you consume, the less the rate of breast cancer. Margarine was found to be detrimental, but no mention was made of this in the body of the article. Apples, bananas, other fruit, broccoli, string beans, cabbage, cauliflower, Brussels sprouts, and carrots all helped to reduce the risk of breast cancer. This also was not mentioned in the original report. There is more. Hot dogs are protective. Also protective are sausage, salami, bologna, bacon, beef, pork, lamb, and even eggs! (The beef, pork, and lamb were only very weakly protective.)

We previously mentioned that cake was said to be protective, but the authors didn't mention the news that cookies are also protective against breast cancer! Even the less exciting cold breakfast cereal is protective. Coffee is also weakly protective against breast cancer. The bad news is that mashed potatoes contribute to breast cancer incidence; rice and pasta do so as well, but only weakly according to the study.

When one carefully dissects this report, it is revealed as a very peculiar piece of work. The problem is that very few physicians, American women, or members of the press seem to have read the article in close detail; nor did more than a handful apparently read the twelve pages of remarkable supplementary material. They were apparently comforted by the names—Harvard, National Institutes of Health, and the American Cancer Society—and looked no further.

Despite the size and the expense of the study, I do not feel that the study design is a proper one. Without a doubt, the number of women in the study *is* large, perhaps too large to be properly handled, especially as we have noted that there was no personal contact with the subjects.

In a study called "Reproducibility of Food Frequency Measurements and Inferences from a Case Control Study," Morabia and others reported on the lack of reliability and accuracy in food measurement and recall when the delay between eating and completing the questionnaire was only *six weeks*.[174] Remember that in the nurses' study the delay was *two years*. The authors conclude that this deficiency may explain discrepant findings in case-control and cohort studies such as the Harvard Nurses' Health Study.

Compare the Harvard study with the data that comes from the Framingham Study headed by Dr. William Castelli. This is a true prospective study. Participants are followed up in person; blood samples are drawn, blood pressure determinations and other verifiable, objective measurements are made, and then conclusions are reached. This honest study design has given us valuable data and lessons for medical practice for more than forty years. The participants are not asked to *estimate* their data, it is *measured* and *verified*.

The Harvard Nurses' Health Study simply reflects the American breast cancer situation as we know it. By this I mean that we already understand that breast cancer is increasing in this country. Simply studying a population at risk without creating a meaningful study group will only confirm what we already know. To learn of the role of fat and fiber in the diet, we must study subgroups of women who will reliably and verifiably undergo significant changes in fat and fiber intake for adequate periods of time starting at a reasonable age. This is the basis of much modern scientific work: a study group that is then compared with a control group.

The study group must be placed on a truly meaningful diet—one that will clearly demonstrate whether or not fat is of consequence. For a true test of the dietary fat/breast cancer link, I would suggest that the percentage of calories as fat be set at not more than 15 percent of total caloric intake. (This would be less than half the current level estimated for American women in general.) The Harvard study claims that the median intake of fat was 33 percent in their 1984 survey. This indicates a possible bias toward underreporting of fat intake by the subjects in the Harvard study. In comparison, a survey of supervised studies, not questionnaires, tells us that the fat intake among the general population of American women—at the time of the study—ranged from 37 to 44 percent of total calories.

Boyar, Rose, and Wynder have reviewed the available experimental and epidemiological evidences and suggest that a diet with fat "as low as 20 percent" of total calories may be necessary to reduce the risk of breast cancer.[175] The authors also performed a feasibility study in premenopausal women with cystic disease and cyclic mastalgia (lumpy breasts and premenstrual breast pain) as well as with postmenopausal women with breast cancer. In three months, the women in the study showed good compliance with a 20-percent-fat diet and *decreases in their serum estrogen levels* were noted. In another 1988 study, Boyar found good patient compliance with dietary modification, and *drops in blood cholesterol* as well as in blood estrogen levels. He recommended cholesterol measurement to verify dietary compliance to the pilot study.[176] There was no similar drop in cholesterol levels reported in the low-fat group of the Harvard Nurses' Study. This is further confirmation that the nurses were not following a diet sufficiently low in fat to protect from breast cancer. Numerous other studies support the feasibility of truly low-fat eating plans for women.[177]

The weight of international epidemiologic studies supports the conclusion that only low levels of fat intake are protective against breast cancer. Breast cancer rates are always low when the intake of fat is 15 percent of calories or less. Remember that the lowest recorded levels of breast cancer are found in societies where the intake of fat is far lower than 20 percent of total calories. The lowest breast cancer rates recorded in China were in a province where the total fat intake was a mere 6 percent of calories. One of the startling findings in Dr. T. Colin Campbell's Cornell-China Study bears repeating. There was no lower threshold for breast cancer protection. In other words, the lower the fat level, the greater the protection. It did not level off at 10 percent, for example. Before you protest that these fat levels are too low and that American women will not adopt such severe diets, please remember that researchers do not perform these scientific studies for purposes of acceptance, compliance, approval, or popularity. Instead, they are designed to establish the truth concerning fat, fiber, and breast cancer. Once that information has been determined, American women will then be able to choose whether or not to follow such a diet. Empowerment requires accurate information. In reference to The Harvard Nurses' Study Barbara Kronman, a codirector of Share, a New York area self-help group for women with breast cancer, had these words: "I think women will be disappointed and will not really believe it. This is one of the few areas in which we can feel some control over our lives. If this gets taken away from us, we are left with a very fatalistic approach."[178]

There are large groups of American women (and men) who happily follow such low-fat diets and strongly prefer them. Their numbers are growing, and you may be surprised to learn that there are already an estimated five to seven million American women who identify themselves as following a very low-fat plan of eating. We have a history in modern American medicine of tempering the very best medical advice with concerns about compliance, acceptability, and popularity with the public. Let's give the public the information and let them decide.

The 1992 Harvard Nurses' Health Study is the second Willett study on breast cancer. The first one was reported in the *New England Journal of Medicine* in 1987.[179] That study had even greater problems than the 1992 Harvard study. One of those problems was the short study period—four years. Another was the narrow range of fat intake (32 to 44 percent of calories). However, the conclusions were exactly the same. Quoting from the 1987 study: "In summary, we found no evidence that total fat intake or consumption of specific types of fat among women was positively associated with the risk of breast cancer." A *Los Angeles Times* science writer commenting on the 1987 article said it very well: "The message on breast cancer prevention continues to be to get the fat out of your food and don't kid yourself with token changes. Cutting from 40 percent to 30 percent is an empty effort. Get to 20 percent at least, by halving your fat intake, bearing in mind where the food fat is: 35 percent of total calories in beef and chicken products, 25 percent in dairy products and 15 percent in the edible oils of dressings, toppings, spreads, fried foods and baked goods." He continued: "Moderate fat reductions are not likely to carry much breast cancer prevention benefit, as several previous population studies demonstrated." I have little to add to that reporter's perceptive analysis.

Can we expect additional studies from Harvard, also assuring us that fat intake and breast cancer are not related, to roll out every four or five years for the next few decades? I strongly suspect so. Each of these will be warmly greeted by the dairy, meat, poultry, and edible-oil industries. More than 160 scientific publications have already emanated from this Harvard cohort of nurses.

When a dietary practice is widespread and considered to be normal, it is highly unlikely to be recognized as important. *Common diseases have common causes.* Yet a so-called normal diet is unlikely to be considered as a cause of cancer. That is why international studies are of such critical importance. They tell us what happens in countries where women have markedly different, lifelong patterns of eating.

It takes many years for the changes in breast cancer incidence fully to unfold among the migrant women mentioned earlier in this book. Breast cancer is a disease resulting, in large part, from a chronic dietary overload in fat and a deficiency in protective plant foods. Studying the genesis of a chronic disease for four years or even the eight years of the Harvard study is too short a time.

For the women of America: take great care in interpreting the 1992 Harvard Nurses' Health Study. If the authors are in error and if you follow their advice, you could pay a terrible price! Although they certainly do not advocate a high-fat diet, they exonerate it as a cause of the most feared of all women's cancers—breast cancer. In a telephone conversation, one of the authors told us, "The evidence is overwhelming that diet is not an important factor in breast cancer. And in any case, American women won't make the change." Look instead at the totality of the world's scientific literature, ponder the above points, and then vote with your knife and fork. It could save your life.

Some of my colleagues feel that I have been too critical of the Harvard Nurses' Health Study. It *is* an important study. It clearly tells us that American women eat too much fat, and it thus confirms the risk of high-fat diets. Several additional valid conclusions were made. First, increasing amounts of dietary fat—even among the heavy users studied—increased the amount of colon cancer encountered; and second, that increasing amounts of ingested alcohol resulted in increasing numbers of breast cancer cases. This information, although not new, confirms the observations of others, and is useful.

It took nearly half a year for a few of the letters of protest from many doctors to be published in the *Journal of the American Medical Association*. This allowed ample time for the information presented initially to solidify in the public's mind prior to any official rebuttal. Dr. Ross Prentice of the Fred Hutchinson Cancer Center in Seattle is a well-known epidemiologist who is coordinating another large study that will look at the health effects of a low-fat diet among American women. "I really don't understand what is happening in that study. I suspect there is a serious methodological problem with the way we're going about diet and cancer studies," said Dr. Prentice. He also wrote a letter subsequently published in the *Journal of the American Medical Association*[180] stating that existing data *already* provides strong evidence for a causal association between fat consumption and postmenopausal breast cancer risk. He felt that the Harvard Nurses' Health Study has such defects that a stronger study design would be necessary to test the hypothesis that "a low-fat eating pattern can prevent breast cancer" among postmenopausal women. He proceeded to outline the inconsistency of results from Willett's Harvard study compared with two other large cohort studies. He described the noteworthy consistency from other data sources, both domestic and foreign, and encouraged Willett and his associates to explore the reasons for their discrepant results. In other words, the Harvard study deviates from the rest of the reputable work in the field, according to Dr. Prentice.

Ernst Wynder, Leonard Cohen, and Steven Stellman of the American Health Foundation of New York also wrote a lengthy letter to the editor of the *Journal of the American Medical Association*, published nearly six months after the October 1992 article.[181] They felt that the conclusions of the Harvard study were unwarranted for the following reasons: First, the study was designed to "test the narrow hypothesis that adult diet measured by a self-administered food questionnaire is related to breast cancer up to 10 years after assessment." Wynder, Cohen, and Stellman felt that the range of dietary exposures within the study was too narrow to provide an adequate test of the critical hypothesis. Ninety percent of the subjects in the study had a total fat intake in excess of 29 percent. Even their lowest "good" group had a median fat intake of 27 percent. Epidemiological and animal studies indicate that the response to fat intake is not linear. A threshold may occur between 20 and 30 percent of calories. This threshold is the level of fat intake below which the cancer-promoting effect of fat is "switched off" and above which it is in full effect. A proper test would require a far wider range of dietary fat ingestion than is usually found in

Western populations of which the nurses are typical. Failure to observe an effect of dietary fat in this study is due to the absence of enough subjects reliably consuming fat below this threshold level. The authors of the letter ended by asking us not to draw conclusions from the results of a single study so flawed by deep methodological and design problems. Instead they asked us to examine the totality of available evidence, which includes half a century of animal-model data, a host of ecological studies, a recent meta-analysis of twelve case-control studies, as well as an analysis of the plausible biological mechanisms, all of which support the dietary fat hypothesis.

*Physician's Weekly* is a nationally distributed, poster-sized periodical that disseminates medical news to most U.S. hospitals. In the April 26, 1993, issue[182] they published a debate: "Is Dietary Fat a Risk Factor for Breast Cancer?" By chance, the proponents of the opposing views were the above-mentioned Dr. Ross L. Prentice and the first coauthor of the Harvard Nurses' Study, Dr. David J. Hunter, assistant professor of epidemiology at the Harvard School of Public Health. It is illuminating to review some of the remarks.

Not surprisingly, Dr. Hunter takes the no position in answer to the question of whether fat is risk factor for breast cancer. Here are some of his views, which are directly quoted from his debate interview in *Physician's Weekly*. I am going to take the liberty of following Dr. Hunter's quoted remarks with my reaction.

Dr. Hunter: "We know enough now to say that at the levels of fat intake prevailing in the U.S., there's unlikely to be any important association between dietary fat and breast cancer."

(*My reaction*: "American women are eating so much fat that nearly all are at risk, they are well above the danger level.")

Dr. Hunter continues: "We still can't exclude the possibility that at very low levels of fat intake—for instance the 15 percent of calories typical of some non-Western diets—there may be a protective effect."

(*My reaction*: "You have indicted your whole study. A 15 percent diet protects billions of women all over the world, and everyone who has studied this subject knows it; the women in your study ate at least twice that much fat.")

Dr. Hunter: "But it would be difficult for women of a Western life-style to achieve that."

(*My reaction*: "Women all over the world can do it, but Dr. Hunter believes that American women are weak-willed and are powerless to save themselves from breast cancer." Such a paternalistic attitude is common among prominent, often elderly, male researchers. One portly and internationally famous expert patted his ample midsection and with a patronizing smile told me, "We can't expect women to change their diets; after all, I can't!" Be wary of this attitude among male policymakers; it can be a danger to your health. Furthermore, I can understand a lack of resolve among American women to make serious lifestyle changes when experts from Harvard tell them that they don't have to change their habits.)

Continuing with Dr. Hunter: "There is indirect evidence though, that fat intake—or more likely total energy intake—during childhood or adolescence may affect risk. Breast cancer rates are low in parts of Asia where many women didn't reach their full potential height, presumably because of calorie restriction during growth, combined perhaps with greater physical activity. But nobody's suggesting that people stunt their children's growth to prevent breast cancer decades later."

(*My reaction*: He's admitting that fat causes breast cancer, but is just haggling over when it does so!)

Nearly sixty years ago, Clive McCay, a researcher at Cornell University, studied rats who were provided a high-fat diet and who then matured early, grew large, developed breast cancers, and died prematurely. We're running the same ghastly experiment with our little girls in the Western nations. Dr. Hunter's use of the phrase *stunt their children's growth* is particularly objectionable. Such wording injects an emotional element that is used to conceal the fault in his argument. No one would intentionally stunt a child's growth. Yet the best evidence shows that the premature and excessive growth following high-fat diets in childhood *will* shorten a child's potential life span. There is no health advantage in oversized children, and pride in an unusually heavy newborn infant is misplaced.[183] The current high rate of cesarean sections in the United States is not an accident; these children are often too large for the normal birth canal. Nutritional influences start in utero! A correct diet not only gives normal stature and avoids gigantism, it protects against breast cancer as well as a number of other diseases.[184]

Dr. Hunter again: "Other prospective studies, though not as large as ours, also found little or no relationship between fat intake and breast cancer."

(*My reaction*: Not so fast, Dr. Hunter! In the same issue of the *Journal of the American Medical Association* as the Harvard Nurses' Study, Dr. Geoffrey R. Howe from the University of Toronto described the Harvard Nurses' Health Study as only one of five such studies. Of the remaining four, three offered evidence to support a positive association between fat intake and breast cancer risk. The fourth was so small—ninety-nine cases—as to be statistically insignificant.[185] Dr. Howe also reports on twelve case-control studies.[186] Nearly all of these also concluded that there *was* a positive association between fat intake and breast cancer risk. Remember, too, that very small differences in large groups can result in large numbers of lives being saved. For example, a risk reduction of only 10 percent of breast cancer patients in the United States could save 18,200 women.

At the annual conference of the American Institute for Cancer Research in Washington, DC, Dr. Hunter was one of five panelists discussing the possible link between dietary fat and breast cancer. Four of the other panelists presented data confirming that a high-fat diet increased the risk of breast cancer. According to a report in *The New York Times* of September 8, 1993, Dr. Hunter was "the only panel member who strongly believed that fat played no role. He suggested that those who believed fat levels had to be lowered to 20 percent to see a difference in breast cancer risk were 'moving the goalposts.' " Dr. Hunter must understand that doctors don't set the goalposts, nature does. It is a bit arrogant to think that we have any control over such a biological matter. Concerning the Harvard Nurses' Health Study, the article says: "To many researchers . . . that study did not compare high-fat and low-fat diets, but high-fat and medium-fat diets." As a result of my concern about the effect of the Harvard study, I also wrote a letter to the editor of the *Journal of the American Medical Association*. Here are some excerpts from my letter:

> This report has done incalculable damage to responsible efforts to reduce the incidence of breast cancer in American women.
>
> Laboratory and human studies have repeatedly demonstrated that levels of fat above 10 percent contribute to an increased incidence of breast cancer. These levels keep rising at 20 percent and top out at 30 percent. There is no evidence that token reductions, say from 40 percent to 30 percent, will be of value. The present study simply confirms these observations.
>
> If American women wish to protect themselves, they should at least halve their fat intake to 20 percent. (Fifteen percent would be better, 10 percent best.) Numerous studies on vegans and religious groups in this

country support this conclusion.

The conclusion reached—'we found no evidence to support the hypothesis that fat intake is a major cause of human breast cancer'—is not warranted by the data published. A more logical and defensible conclusion would be: 'All American women consuming the standard American diet are at nearly equal risk. They must substantially reduce the amount of ingested fat to reach the protective levels that international studies clearly teach us.' Students of breast cancer epidemiology understand that these international data clearly and consistently show protection only when the total fat level is *20 percent of calories or less*. Should women migrate from protected countries to a country with a high breast cancer rate and adopt the diet of that society, their breast cancer rates sharply increase. There have been no exceptions in nearly a dozen such migration studies.

Finally, articles such as this one lead to cynicism and confusion as women are first told that their risk of breast cancer can be reduced by dietary means, and then are told that there is no connection between the two. Major dietary changes are required and should be recommended. Moderate reductions are known to be ineffective, this study confirms it.

I received a courteous letter from the editors of the *Journal of the American Medical Association* telling me that they simply had too many letters to print and not enough space. I couldn't help but notice that two of the four letters that they did publish concerning the Harvard Nurses' Health Study seemed flimsy, with no direct or challenging assertions. One questioned the protective role of cigarette smoking, and the other discussed the effect of alcohol. It is easy to defend oneself when you can pick your own questions and take many months to compose your answers.

Do these nine researchers truly believe that fat has nothing to do with breast cancer as they so clearly say? Are they unconvinced by the many studies that have produced opposite results? Are they incapable of perceiving the defects in their methodology? Are they untroubled by their aberrant conclusions?

My analysis of the Harvard Nurses' Health Study is provided to help you to clarify your thinking about what is possibly the most important woman's health issue of the decade. We will next focus on the issue of funding for research.

# ∞ Appendix 2

## Research Funding:
## An Incentive for Bias?

W ho sponsored the Harvard Nurses' breast cancer study? And for that matter, why should we care? Because American women need to know if the health information that they receive is *free from bias*. At issue is the funding of university studies and university researchers by interested food-industry groups. Such funding could clearly result in pressure on those investigators to deliver conclusions that are acceptable to the sponsors, should the investigators hope to continue receiving funds from those sponsors.

The Harvard Nurses' Health Study officially lists as its sponsors the National Institutes of Health (two grants), and one of the authors was supported by a grant from the American Cancer Society, both institutions of the highest repute.

Shortly after the publication of the *Journal of the American Medical Association* article, my office called the National Institutes of Health (NIH) and asked about other sources of funding, and specifically about food-industry funding for the Harvard Nurses' Health Study. They declined to give me funding information, but instead told me a number of times that they "were not required to reveal private sources of funding," and that "We are prevented by law from revealing private sources of funding." At no time did they deny the existence of private funding, they only denied access to the identity of those providing it.

After many fruitless telephone calls, we finally contacted the Freedom of Information Office at the NIH. A pleasant woman repeated the message about not being allowed to divulge private sources of funding, but at my insistence she did ship me a large package of documents that were alleged to contain information—revealed only under the Freedom of Information Act—concerning funding sources. I dutifully plowed through this huge pile of documents, one by one. There was no clue about any private funding.

Upon further request, a second large package of documents arrived in January of 1993 with the same results, no information about private sources of funding. Also included was a great deal of irrelevant information concerning unrelated studies on lung diseases, diabetes, etc. By this time one of the authors had been told of our inquiries and called us, asking about our interest in the study and the grants. When questioned about food-industry sponsorship, he at first said there was none, but much later in the conversation did admit that the dairy industry was involved in "another part" of the study.

We next sent a letter to the NIH Freedom of Information Office protesting the lack of meaningful information concerning possible food-industry funding for the Harvard Nurses' Health Study. We received a response on April 21, 1993, from Joanne Belk, acting Freedom of Information officer at the NIH. Here is a portion of her reply: "I have determined to withhold that information under the provisions of 5 U.S.C. 552 (b) (4) and (6) of the Act and 45 CFR 5.65 and 5.67 of the Regulation. Exemption 4 is intended to protect commercial or financial information obtained from a person which is privileged or confidential. Exemption 6 exempts from disclosure information that would cause a clearly unwarranted invasion of personal privacy. You have a right to appeal this decision to deny you access to records in the Agency's possession."

Consider the reasons for denial: commercial or financial interests, and personal privacy. In our opinion, none of these concerns is remotely reasonable. The "Freedom of Information" Office at the NIH is unable or unwilling to answer the simple question: "Is the food industry involved in the funding of the Harvard Nurses' Health Study?" We appealed their decision to withhold the information. The appeal was denied.

Can you imagine the frustration of an interested American woman who might wish to know if the information she was receiving was potentially biased? The exercise described above took hours of a staffer's time, a considerable amount of money for telephone calls, a modest amount of money for copying fees, and a great deal of persistence.

We persisted, appealed the denial, and was again rejected. We have not tried further. The final denial came directly from the newly appointed assistant secretary for health, Philip R. Lee, M.D., and was dated August 25, 1993. Dr. Lee was the former chancellor of the University of California Medical School at San Francisco, and was also an assistant secretary for health in the Johnson administration twenty-six years earlier. In his letter, he provided additional irrelevant funding information, but said: "I must continue to deny you access to the private funding deleted from the grants. This information is considered confidential financial information submitted by the grantee. We have no discretion to disclose it." And: "Because this denial constitutes final agency action, you may seek review in the District Court of the United States in the district in which you reside."

We were told by his staffers that Dr. Lee carefully reviewed the entire request and file prior to writing the letter.

"Don't make a federal case out of it!" is usually spoken in exasperation when someone inappropriately makes a very large issue out of a small one. I feel that is exactly what has happened here. I asked a reasonable and highly appropriate question: "Is the food industry involved in an important study that centers directly on both food and women's health?" The potential for introduction of bias is obvious to all. We were told after nearly a year of persistent probing literally to "make a federal case out of it" and to seek further remedy in the district court of the United States.

The total payoff to date: only a verbal acknowledgment from one of the authors that the dairy industry is involved in "some part of the study." I have abandoned my attempts to learn of food-industry involvement in the Harvard Nurses' Health Study. It may seem tedious to relate these events in detail, but the reason for doing so is to demonstrate the levels of concealment on behalf of private donors, whoever they may be.

A similar question was posed to the editors of the *Nurses' Health Study Newsletter* in June 1993. The question was: "How is this study funded?" The answer: "Most of our funding is provided by grants from the National Cancer Institute, the National Institutes of Health (NIH), and from other federal agencies." The NIH admits that there *is* private funding in addition to their funding, but state that they are prohibited by law from divulging the sources of that funding.

Relationships between the academic world and industry were explored in a special communication from the *Journal of the American Medical Association* on December 16, 1992.[187] The author is from the Health Policy Research and Development Unit of the Massachusetts General Hospital and the Harvard Medical School. Although much of the article centers on devices and drugs that have proprietary value, there is also attention given to "concerns that health care research sometimes involves patients whose welfare might conceivably be compromised in the service of the business interests of investigators and industries." One of the five types of relationships is described as "the support by industry (through grant or contract) of university-based research." In 1985, a Harvard project on university–industry relationships found that of eight hundred faculty who responded, 47 percent consulted to industry. Even 19 percent of seven hundred graduate students received research or educational support from industries. The author of this *Journal of the American Medical Society* study felt that the two most important lessons about the risks of industry–academic relations was that "the real or apparent conflicts of interest created by Academic Industry Relationships can be damaging to the public reputation of the health sciences, even when no misconduct or even any bias can be documented." The second lesson was that "involvement of the life sciences in clinical research creates special responsibilities for health care researchers and special risks for their AIRs [academic–industry relationships]. Even more than colleagues in other fields, investigators whose research may affect the health of their human subjects have an ethical obligation to avoid potential biases that economic conflicts of interest may create."[188]

The government tried to solve this problem with no success. In September 1989, the National Institutes of Health proposed guidelines concerning conflicts of interest. These guidelines were met with vigorous protests from both the academic institutions and the industries. The guidelines were quickly withdrawn. All parties are still working on a compromise.

The Congress of the United States has a Subcommittee on Oversight and Investigations, with Congressman John D. Dingell of Michigan as the chairman. In the June 3, 1993, *New England Journal of Medicine*[189] Congressman Dingell describes his committee's findings on misconduct in medical research. It is a chilling tale of fraud, plagiarism, fabrications, and embezzlement. One of the first cases that the committee considered was that of a researcher who committed an act of fraud. Quoting from Congressman Dingell's writing: "Two investigations were conducted at the medical school—the first by Dr. X's immediate supervisor and department chairman, and the second by a committee of faculty members from Harvard and elsewhere that the dean had appointed. Both reported no misconduct in X's published research. A third committee, appointed by the NIH, discovered a massive fraud; the data for Dr. X's published experiments did not exist. This was particularly awkward for Harvard, which had maintained up to that point that its investigators had reviewed the data fully—the same data that later turned out not to exist." This unpleasant matter is reviewed not to condemn a university, but to illustrate that these problems can occur at any level. Even the massive National Surgical Adjuvant Breast Program was plagued by reports of falsified data from a Canadian researcher in 1994, resulting in the resignation of the project director.

Another Harvard professor has placed himself on record as opposing any interference in funding. In a remarkable article entitled "Conflict of Interest, the New McCarthyism in Science," Kenneth J. Rothman makes the following assertions published in the *Journal of the American Medical Association*.[190] He is opposed to policies that require authors to disclose potential conflicts of interest on the basis that "disclosure policies would allow readers to make a more informed and therefore better interpretation of published work." Dr. Rothman states that "informed judgment is not always better judgment." He continues, "A conflict of interest by itself does not indicate wrongdoing—it merely refers to a setting in which factors exist that might influence one's conduct. Not everyone subjected to the temptation of placing his or her self-interest above responsibility to others succumbs to that temptation. Journals could simply ask authors to disclose how objective they think they are. Cynics would argue that authors cannot be objective about assessing their own objectivity, so their responses would not be useful. It is also easier to lie about one's objectivity than one's financial ties, for which records usually exist. For these reasons, asking directly about objectivity might not have a high enough sensitivity in detecting biased work to satisfy zealots." If you are more reassured by looking at financial records than taking someone's word that they are honest, Dr. Rothman might label you a zealot! In view of the sorry record of theft, bias, misrepresentation, and outright lying that has, on occasion, appeared in our scientific journals, I suggest that we all become zealots immediately. In my opinion, industry should not support research; in the end, the American public pays too dearly.

If information concerning possible conflict of interest reaches the reader, Dr. Rothman worries about the outcome: "Exactly how is this information to be put to use? . . . Some say that we should use the information by directing more intense scrutiny toward papers written by suspect authors who might be subject to 'conflicts'." He next makes the remarkable leap that this will lead to "irrationalism" by steering us away from judging a work on its merits and says, "Lofty motives notwithstanding, when readers are urged to judge a work by the source of funding, the sexual orientation of the investigator, the investigator's religious beliefs, and other such consideration, irrationalism is the end result."

Notice how two bogus issues are mixed together with a real issue to lead to an unwarranted conclusion. No fair person ever discriminates on the basis of sexual orientation or religious belief. But at the same time, no discerning person would ever disregard the source of funding. There is a world of difference between the two, and I resent the implications made in lumping them together. Dr. Rothman goes on to say that "readers may judge a work by the reputation of the author or institution where the work was done. Thus, one could argue that publication should be anonymous." I don't consider this a reasoned and critical statement from an academic leader. He concludes that "it seems unnecessary to have disclosures become a mandatory part of the review process."

The problem of industry funding has been discussed extensively in medical journals. Here are some sample quotations from an article "Medicine at Center Stage" that appeared in the April 29, 1993, *New England Journal of Medicine*, written by the editor in chief of that journal, Jerome P. Kassirer, M.D.[191] "Universities and academic medical centers must develop clear standards that define what is and what is not an appropriate academic-industrial relationship for their institutions and faculties, insist that their investigators reveal all their relations to industry, and proscribe direct conflicts of interest." Elsewhere in his editorial he says that many people now reject the definition of conflict of interest as simply the appearance of such a conflict or even the actual behavior based on bias. They now believe that "A more widely accepted and stringent criterion is whether there is an incentive for bias; if there is, then a conflict of interest exists whether or not anyone succumbs to the temptation. We have also come to understand that the mere disclosure of a conflict of interest . . . is not an acceptable way out."

Dr. Kassirer's predecessor as editor at the *New England Journal of Medicine* was Arnold S. Relman, M.D. Dr. Relman is now the emeritus Editor-in-Chief. In an editorial on April 6, 1989,[192] he also lamented the increasing commercialization of medicine, but went on:

Like medical practice, medical research is also becoming commercialized, and clinical investigators now find themselves in situations involving similar conflicts of interest . . . they may be receiving support for their laboratory from the company . . . Clinical investigators as well as practicing physicians have an obligation to make unbiased professional judgments, uninfluenced by personal financial interests . . . Economic incentives can introduce subtle biases into the conduct, analysis, or reporting of research results that may escape even careful peer review. Such incentives can also bias review articles and public statements about their work, which in turn may have important effects on the clinical decisions of practicing physicians. Later work by others will probably correct any errors resulting from these biases but not before damage has been done by the dissemination of misleading clinical information. My primary objection to financial ties of this kind is that they erode scientific objectivity and engender the loss of public trust . . . Whatever is done should be discussed collectively and in public. Leaving arrangements to the private discretion of individual researchers and companies will surely multiply problems that are already receiving unfavorable public attention.

## The Harvard Department of Nutrition and Dr. Fredrick J. Stare

The Nurses' Health Study came from the Harvard Department of Nutrition. Let's trace the history of this department in relation to the food industry. Judge for yourself whether it meets the standards outlined by Dr. Kassirer. The department was founded in 1942, and at first received funds from the federal government. However, those funds declined in 1945 as the war was coming to an end. Generous research grants from the National Institutes of Health had not yet begun. What to do?

The founder of the Harvard Department of Nutrition,

and its chairman for thirty-four years, is a remarkable gentleman by the name of Dr. Fredrick J. Stare. By all accounts he is a charming and able individual who has certainly made an indelible impression on nutritional teaching not only in America but around the world. Here is the story of the founding of the Harvard Department of Nutrition—the source of the Harvard Nurses' Health Study—as told by Dr. Fredrick J. Stare, Ph.D., M.D., in his fascinating autobiography, *Adventures in Nutrition*, published in 1991.[193] Of initial interest is a bold-print blurb on the back of the book jacket. Here is precisely what it says: "Of particular interest to contemporary nutritionists are Dr. Stare's 'tips' on fund raising, particularly private funds, for both research and teaching. This requires long cultivation with patience, persistence and politeness."

Pondering a source of funds for the then cash-poor department of nutrition at Harvard in the 1940s, he found the food industry a logical source of private funds for support of such studies. Dr. Stare continues:

My father was president of a large vegetable canning company with several factories in Wisconsin, Indiana, and Kansas . . . through him I was able to meet the 'top men' in several major food companies. My major effort was to convince these leaders of the food industry that they should be willing to provide unrestricted funds for support of basic research in the science of nutrition and in nutrition education for the public and the health professions. Soon we began to get unrestricted grants varying in size from $2,500 to $10,000, not large gifts today, but sizable in the late 1940s and 1950s . . . When one of my top contacts was about to retire or move on to another position, I made sure that he would introduce me to his successor.

I thought that writing for the public was part of our

responsibility in a School of Public Health to educate the public in good nutrition and counteract the nonsense of the food faddists and health food enthusiasts who were as prevalent then as they are today. These writings were also very helpful in raising funds.

Not too many chief executive officers of food or pharmaceutical companies read these magazines, but I would send them a copy of our piece with a brief note suggesting they take it home to their wives, and I would always end these notes with: 'Let me know whenever I might be helpful to you.' That last sentence was paramount in gaining goodwill. I was pleasantly surprised at how often I was asked for suggestions on a personal or family health problem. I firmly believe that over the years this was an effective way to 'cultivate' the top people in the food industry and thus have them continue to provide us with unrestricted funds.

I see the food supply of America as a source of not only nourishment, but also as a dangerous and potent source of disease. Dr. Stare seems to see it as the embodiment of near perfection on the part of the food industry, distorted only by poor food choices on the part of consumers, and the antics of diet faddists and "quacks" such as myself.

Dr. Stare continues in *Adventures in Nutrition*:

National Dairy increased their unrestricted contributions to us and when we needed funds for a new building in the early 1960s, they joined several other companies in making contributions of $100,000 each

Dr. Stare writes:.

Another round of cultivation which resulted in substantial grants to the Department over a period of years involved Lever Brothers, the American subsidiary of Unilever, the huge Anglo-Dutch Company that operates all over the world and is one of the largest manufacturers of margarines, cooking fats, and oils . . . We needed a special margarine, high in polyunsaturates, and not then available, for studies with about 400 adolescent boys in a boarding school . . . Not only did they supply all the margarine for this two-year study, but they also contributed generous amounts of unrestricted funds to the Department. A couple of years after this study, the specially prepared margarine was on the market under the name of *Promise.*

I must add that the development of margarines is hardly a development to be proud of. The world gets a margarine, and Harvard gets money; is this a good arrangement? Current understanding is that margarines are definitely not health-promoting foodstuffs. The output from his former institution's *Nurses' Health Study Newsletter,* June 1993, supports this: "Women with a consistently high level of margarine intake over a 10-year period had a 67% increase in the risk of CHD." (CHD represents coronary heart disease.)

Dr. Stare: "Luckily for me, in 1960, I was elected a director of the Continental Can Company. . . . This directorship opened an entirely new set of important business contacts . . . But my best tale of luck concerns the late Mr. John A. Hartford . . . . Mr. John . . . and his brother, George L. Hartford, had inherited the A&P from their father who started the company. They had built it into the largest supermarket company in the world." In a meeting, Dr. Stare told John Hartford that he "hoped we could interest food manufacturers and individuals who had become wealthy from the food industry to help support us." He was given only $2,000. ". . . I made a point of writing Mr. Hartford a half-page letter about every other month, not asking for more money, but mentioning the activities of the Department and those food industries that were beginning to support us and the size of their grants which were then in the range of $5,000 to $10,000." Mr. Hartford unexpectedly died but had established an endowment to Dr. Stare's department of nutrition of $200,000 yearly for ten years. His company also supplied an additional $843,291.

Dr. Stare cultivated two other Endowment Funds: The James E. Knox Memorial Fund for Nutrition Education and the Nutrition Education Fund. The Knox Fund was related to the Knox Gelatin Co. As of June 30, 1990, it had a balance of $249,582 and produced an income of $20,933.

In 1976, Dr. Stare was required to resign his Department chairmanship by long-standing Harvard rules, but his involvement in the Department of Nutrition continued. Along with continuing to raise an average of $200,000 annually in private funds, he felt a continuing responsibility to those who had given private funds to the Department, including the Trustees of the Stare Fund, to see that the funds are used for purposes for which they were given. Dr. Stare noted that "private donors . . . provided 80 percent of the funds for the nutrition laboratories." These comments clearly indicate that Dr. Stare felt an obligation to the donors and their desires, and thus their gifts were not truly unrestricted and without conditions.

Dr. Stare, as emeritus professor, became involved in the issue of food labeling; in so doing, he gives us a clear indication of his approach to consumer information. In a letter, dated June 29, 1990, to senior group director, Community and Economic Division, U.S. General Accounting Office, concerning a proposed food-labeling regulation, Dr. Stare said that the labeling "would not be used or understood by most consumers," and "If the present administration is interested in reducing government expenses, they could well ask FDA and USDA to forgo extensive nutritional labeling for a few more years. . . . On the other hand, nutrition education *via advertising* is important." [my emphasis] Dr. Stare apparently feels that the public is too lazy or dull to perceive the information in accurate food labeling and should instead receive their "nutritional education" by way of food-industry advertising. As a consumer, I am very interested in precise nutritional labeling. I know that I'm not alone in this, either.

In a July 2, 1990, letter to Dr. James O. Mason, assistant secretary of health and human services, Dr. Stare said, "To me, extensive nutritional labeling is pretty much a waste of time and money. . . . Why go to the trouble and expense of labeling them except to satisfy the whims of a few noisy consumer activists."

People closely reading labels clog the aisles of supermarkets in my area. A large segment of society is intensely interested in the food that they take into their own bodies or provide for those they love.

Dr. Stare later took his own view of "consumer activism" to the chief of staff for then President George Bush, Governor John H. Sunnunu. Writing in opposition to the book *Diet for a Poisoned Planet* by David Steinman[194] Dr. Stare described a central thesis of the book as "that many foods . . . including milk chocolate, peanut butter, cheese, and ice cream, contain dangerously high levels of toxins and pesticides. This statement is false! We have by far the safest food supply of any country, and our FDA and USDA help keep it that way. It would be helpful if you and others in the Bush administration would speak out on these issues." Now that is trying to help your friends! Here we have the most respected nutritionist in America, an emeritus professor from Harvard, appealing to the highest level in a United States president's administration on behalf of his old friends and benefactors.

Dr. Stare is seemingly not concerned about the *trans*-fatty acids, either. In a letter to the acting director, Office of

Nutrition and Food Sciences, FDA, Washington, DC, he said, "Ever since hydrogenated fats came into general use, some 30 to 40 years ago, death from coronary heart disease has decreased, a total of approximately 30 percent . . . I think we should have a better try at improving nutrition education of the public at all ages and walks of life before we spend more time and money on more extensive food labeling."

We also must be fair and evaluate Dr. Stare in connection with his time. When he first appealed to the food industry for funding in the period following World War II, there was virtually no awareness of hazard in our daily food. However, when this information gradually became available in the mid-1950s and later, his tone of uncritical adulation did not seem to change.

Here is an example of this support quoted from his 1989 book, *Balanced Nutrition Beyond the Cholesterol Scare*, written with two former staff members.[195] "We wrote this book to address the unfounded concerns many people have about the safety and quality of the American food supply. Today, many of us are alarmed when we hear the word 'cholesterol' in connection with our diets. . . . The reality is that our food supply is the best, safest, and most nutritious of any in the world. The government agencies charged with overseeing this high quality are, on the whole, doing an excellent job. . . . We believe many of the most prestigious medical organizations in the country have made ill-advised and irresponsible decisions on a number of important contemporary health issues."

I fear that the thinking Dr. Stare and his coauthors dismiss may often represent the work of thoughtful persons, correctly and appropriately warning us about serious problems in our food supply. Dr. Stare continues, "Diet changes may be advisable for high-risk individuals in an attempt to reduce their risk factors for certain diseases (specifically coronary heart disease), but such changes are not, in our opinion, warranted for the entire U.S. population." This statement was written in an era when the fat consumption averaged over 40 percent of all calories. Doesn't this advice really sound more like the recommendation of a food-industry spokesman than the considered medical advice of the world's leading nutritionist?

Dr. Stare's department at Harvard gave a huge "gift" back to the food industry: the "basic-four food groups." Concerning those four food groups, Dr. Stare says: "The USDA adopted them in 1957, but made no mention that they originated from Harvard's Department of Nutrition two years earlier!" The basic-four food groups, in case someone was dozing in school, are made up of meats, milk and dairy products, cereal grains, and fruits and vegetables. While this superficially sounds acceptable, and certainly one can make a good diet out of the four groups, there is a great deal wrong with the four food group concept. It gives the strong impression that these groups are of equal importance. They certainly are not. There is abundant evidence that if the meat and dairy groups were removed, or at least greatly reduced, from our adult diets, we would be immensely better off. Even growing children are given far too much fat and protein. Millions of dollars have been spent by the food industry in fostering and perpetuating the four-food-group concept. Who among us has not seen the glossy, large charts in the schoolroom colorfully depicting the four food groups? However, very few of us have peered at the bottom edge of those charts to learn that they were provided by members of the food industry. The damage to the health of America caused by the nutritional distortions of the four food group concept is impossible to estimate. So are the profits to the food industry.

On April 28, 1992, Secretary of Agriculture Edward R. Madigan released the new USDA food pyramid replacing the old four food groups. This was not accomplished without a spirited fight from the meat and dairy industries, who delayed it and remain opposed to it on the basis that it gives the image of "good foods and bad foods." They also did not like the position of meat on the pyramid chart. The food pyramid is not perfect. For example, it groups beans with meat, poultry, fish, eggs, and nuts. Clearly the beans are far lower in fat and should be given a more favorable position. However, the pyramid is a definite improvement over the unbalanced four food groups.

Do not underestimate the impact of the Harvard Department of Nutrition and Dr. Stare. The graduates from the Harvard Department of Nutrition have become heads of most of the nutritional departments in this country. Thousands of advanced students have disseminated from the Department of Nutrition. The impact of these graduates has been, and continues to be, enormous. If Dr. Stare's nutritional viewpoints are colored by his stated, lifelong, and close bonds with the food industry, and those views are even partially accepted by his students who are now our professors— the damage to our country, and perhaps some of the rest of the world, will be difficult to assess.

Dr. Stare is reassured, however. The reason? He finally has a successor that he is satisfied with in Dr. Walter C. Willett who became Chairman of the Department of Nutrition in 1991 after being recommended by Dr. Stare.

At present, Dr. Willett is the "Fredrick John Stare Professor of Epidemiology and Nutrition."

So now the circle is closed; Dr. Stare, who admits that the food industry gave him over $20 million (worth many times more than this in today's dollars), and who simply cannot find it in himself to say anything negative about his benefactors, has named his successor, Walter Willett, author of the Harvard Nurses' Health Study. Will Dr. Willett follow the same course as Dr. Stare? We know for a fact that the Harvard Department of Nutrition in the past received large infusions of money from the food industries. We now also clearly understand that many of the foods produced by these very sponsors can contribute to our most serious diseases, chiefly heart disease, cancer, and stroke. Will these Harvard investigators continue to assure American women every four years that dietary fat has nothing to do with breast cancer? If you accept money from the food industry, are you entirely free to tell the truth about their products? It seems that appropriate criticism of our food supply is unlikely to come from research institutes heavily supported by food-industry money.

The issue is clear. Much of our highly varied, desired, and profitable food supply has been found to be dangerous. The people who furnish this food and who are enriched by its sale do not want you to know this. They have generously contributed to scientists who have supported, and are willing to continue to support, their products. If those scientists suddenly have a change of heart, and seriously challenge the safety of that food, you may be certain that the bulk of the food-industry financial support will promptly disappear.

Whom are you going to believe? Those with no financial gain from the sale of food and with the backing of the world's scientific literature? Or are you going to follow those who have at times devised flawed studies and reaped millions of dollars in support from the industries that they fail to seriously criticize? You must decide, and your health will be substantially determined by your decision.

Here is a *partial* listing from Dr. Stare's autobiography, *Adventures in Nutrition,* of companies in the food and pharmaceutical industries that have contributed to the Harvard Department of Nutrition and the research laboratories. Read it carefully. This is listed under "Gifts from industry, 1942 to 1990."

The "lead gift" of $1,026,000 was from General Foods. In alphabetical order: Abbott Laboratories, Allied Supermarkets, American Meat Institute, Armour and Co., Beatrice

Food Co., Beechnut Packing Co., Bird's Eye—Division of General Foods Corporation, Borden Co. Foundation, California Hawaiian Sugar Co., California Packing Corp., Campbell Institute for Food Research, Campbell Soup Co., Carnation Co., Cereal Institute., Coca-Cola Co., Continental Can Co., Corn Products Co., Council for Tobacco Research, Dairy Council of California, Finn-Cal Fruit Sugar Co., Frito-Lay, Inc., General Mills, Gerber Baby Food Company, Great Atlantic and Pacific Tea Co., Grocery Manufacturers of America, H. J. Heinz Co. Foundation., Hershey Foods, Hoffman La-Roche, Hunt-Wesson Foods, International Sugar Research Foundation, Junket Brand Foods, Kellogg Company, Kraft Corp, Lever Brothers Co., Eli Lilly & Co., Thomas J. Lipton Foundation, Maine Sardine Council, Marion Laboratories, Oscar Mayer Co., Maxwell House—Division of General Foods, McDonald's Corp., Minute Maid Corp., Monsanto Co., National Biscuit Co., National Canners Association., National Confectioners Association, National Dairy Council, National Dairy Products, National Livestock & Beef Board, National Vitamin Foundation, Nestlé Coordination Center for Nutrition, Inc., Parke, Davis & Co., Pepsico Foundation, Inc., Pet Milk Co., Pillsbury Co., Quaker Oats Co., Safeway Stores, Inc., Special Dairy Industry Board, Standard Brands, Star-Kist Foods, Inc., Sucrest Corporation, Sugar Association, Inc., Sugar Research Foundation, Swift and Company Foundation, Tobacco Industries Research Foundation, Tropicana Products, Tuna Research Foundation, Wheat Flour Institute, and many others not listed here. In addition to this listing, Dr. Stare offers another list of private donors also from 1942 to 1990. These include Oscar G. Mayer, Jr., the Nutrition Foundation, Vernon Stouffer, and the Nestlé Foundation.

# Chapter Notes

**CHAPTER 1    BREAST CANCER: THE NEGLECTED EPIDEMIC**

[1] C. C. Boring et al, Cancer Statistics, *CA: A Cancer Journal for Clinicians*, 44:1 (January/February 1994), p. 19.

[2] A. I. Holleb, D. J. Fink and G. P. Murphy, *Textbook of Clinical Oncology*, Atlanta, GA, American Cancer Society, 1991, p. 2.

[3] L. Garfinkel, "Evaluating Cancer Statistics," *CA: A Cancer Journal for Clinicians*, 44:1 (January/February 1994), p. 6.

[4] J. G. Klijn et al, "Clinical breast cancer, new developments in selection and endocrine treatment of patients," *Journal of Steroid Biochemistry and Molecular Biology*, 43:1–3 (September 1992), pp. 21–221.

[5] C. B. Mueller, F. Ames and G. D. Anderson, "Breast cancer in 3,558 women—Age as a significant determinant in the rate of dying and causes of death," *Surgery*, 83:2 (February 1978), pp. 12–132.

[6] D. Plotkin and F. Blankenberg, "Breast cancer—biology and malpractice," *American Journal of Clinical Oncology*, 14: 3 (1991), pp. 254–266.

[7]L. E. Rutqvist, A. Wallgren and B. Nilsson, "Is breast cancer a curable disease? A study of 14,731 women with breast cancer from the cancer registry of Norway," *Cancer*, 53 (1984), pp. 1793–1800.

[8]A. O. Langlands et al, "Longterm survival of patients with breast cancer: a study of the curability of the disease," *British Medical Journal*, 2 (1979), pp. 1247–1251.

[9]D. Brinkley and J. L. Haybittle, "Long-term survival of women with breast cancer," *Lancet*, 1 (May 19, 1984), p. 1118.

[10]L. Garfinkel, "Current trends in breast cancer," *CA: A Cancer Journal for Clinicians*, 43:1 (January/February 1993), p. 5.

[11]M. R. Spitz, "Cancer Prevention," in *Mosby Year Book*, St. Louis, Missouri, M. D. Anderson Cancer Center, 1992, p. 21.

[12]G. E. Dinse and D. G. Hoel, "Exploring time trends in cancer research," *Journal of Cancer Causes and Control*, 3:5 (September 1992), pp. 409–417.

[13]T. R. Holford et al, "Trends in female breast cancer in Connecticut and the United States," *Journal of Clinical Epidemiology*, 44:1 (1991), pp. 29–39.

[14]A. G. Glass and R. N. Hoover, "Rising incidence of breast cancer: relationship to stage and receptor status," *Journal of the National Cancer Institute*, 18:82(8) (April 18, 1990), pp. 693–696.

[15]G. A. Colditz et al, "Family history, age, and risk of breast cancer," *Journal of the American Medical Association*, 270: 3 (July 21, 1993), pp. 338–343.

[16]J. A. Mayer et al, "Evaluation of a media-based mammography program," *American Journal of Preventive Medicine*, *8:1* (January 1992), pp. 23–29.

## CHAPTER 2   HOW BREAST CANCER BEGINS:
## CURRENT BELIEFS

[17]J. M. Bishop, "Genes Gone Awry," in *Cancer Today*, ed. L. Roberts, Washington, DC, National Academy Press, (1984).

[18]B. B. Biesecker, "Genetic counseling for families with inherited susceptibility to breast and ovarian cancer," *Journal of the American Medical Association,* 269:15 (April 21, 1993), pp. 1970–1974.

[19]D. I. W. Phillips, "Twin studies in medical research: can they tell us whether diseases are genetically determined?" *Lancet,* 341 (April 17, 1993), pp. 1008–1009.

[20]T. I. A. Sorensen et al, "Genetic and environmental influences on premature death in adult adoptees," *New England Journal of Medicine,* 318:12 (March 24, 1988), pp. 727–732.

[21]G. A. Colditz et al, "Family history, age, and risk of breast cancer," *Journal of the American Medical Association,* 270: 3 (October 6, 1993), pp. 338–343.


## CHAPTER 3   PREVENTION IS THE ANSWER

[22]William B. Walsh, *Hope in the East: the Mission to Ceylon,* New York: E. P. Dutton, (1970).

[23]*USA Today,* August 25, 1993.


## CHAPTER 5   THE DIET CONNECTION: THE EVIDENCE

[24]E. L. Wynder et al, "Clinical trials of dietary interventions to enhance cancer survival," in *Recent Progress in Research on Nutrition and Cancer,* New York, Wiley-Liss Inc., (1990), pp. 217–229.

[25]E. Taioli et al, "Dietary habits and breast cancer: a comparative study of United States and Italian data," *Nutrition and Cancer,* 16:3–4 (1991), pp. 259–265.

[26]B. Bjerregaard and A. Kung'u, "Breast cancer in Kenya: a histopathologic and epidemiologic study," *East African Medical Journal,* 69:1 (January 1991), pp. 22–26.

[27]S. K. Gupta et al, "Breast Cancer in Papua, New Guinea: a survey of 10 years," *Australia and New Zealand Journal of Surgery,* 60:1 (January 1990), pp. 41–44.

[28]T. Colin Campbell, *A Study on Diet, Nutrition and Disease in the People's Republic of China*, Ithaca, New York: Cornell University Press, (1990).

[29]E. L. Wynder et al, "Comparative epidemiology of cancer between the United States and Japan," *Cancer*, 67 (1991), pp. 746–785.

[30]Y. Kagawa, "Impact of Westernization on the nutrition of Japanese," *Preventive Medicine*, 7 (1978), pp. 205–217.

[31]E. L. Wynder et al, "Comparative epidemiology of cancer between the United States and Japan. A second look," *Cancer*, 67 (February 1, 1991), pp. 746–763.

[32]Stuart J. Schnitt et al, "The increasing prevalence of benign proliferative breast lesions in Japanese women," *Cancer*, 71:8 (April 15, 1993), pp. 2528–2531.

[33]R. R. Love, Personal communication with Richard R. Love, Professor Oncology, University of Wisconsin, Madison, Wisconsin. At Conference: *Controversies in Breast Cancer 1993 September 11, 1993, San Francisco, California.*

[34]United States Department of Agriculture, "Nutrient content of the U.S. food supply," *Human Nutrition Information Service Administration Report 229–21*, Hyattsville, MD, (1988), pp. 8–9.

[35]L. J. Vatten, K. Sovall, and E. B. Loken, "Frequency of meat and fish intake and risk of breast cancer in a prospective study of 14,500 Norwegian women," *International Journal of Cancer*, 15:46 (July 1990), pp. 12–15.

[36]K. Sugiura, *The Publications of Kanematsu Sugiura: Memorial Edition*, 4 volumes, foreword by Chester Stock, New York: Sloan-Kettering Institute, (1965).

[37]C. L. Meschter, J. M. Connolly and D. P. Rose, "Influence of regional location of the inoculation site and dietary fat on the pathology of MDA-MB-435 human breast cancer cell-derived tumors grown in nude mice," *Clinical and Experimental Metastasis*, 10:3 (May 1992), pp. 167–173.

[38]E. M. Scholar et al, "The effect of diets enriched in cabbage and collards on murine pulmonary metastasis," *Nutrition and Cancer*, 12:2 (1989), pp. 121–126.

[39]H. Gabor et al, "Effect of dietary fat and monoclonal antibody therapy on the growth of human mammary adenocarcinoma MX-1 grafted in athymic mice," *Cancer Letters*, 52:3 (July 31, 1990), pp. 173–178.

[40]M. Noguchi et al, "Effects of switching from a high-fat diet to a low-fat diet on tumor proliferation and cell kinetics of 7, 12-dimethylbenz (a) anthracene-induced mammary carcinoma in rats," *Oncology*, 49:3 (1992), pp. 246–252.

[41]Z. Djuric et al, "Effects of a low-fat diet on levels of oxidative damage to DNA in human peripheral nucleated blood cells," *Journal of the National Cancer Institute*, 83:11 (June 5, 1991), pp. 766–769.

[42]K. Carroll, "Dietary fat in relation to tumorigenesis," *Progress in Biochemical Pharmacology*, 10 (1975), pp. 308–353.

[43]J. Barone, "Dietary fat and natural killer-cell activity," *American Journal of Clinical Nutrition*, 50 (1989), pp. 861–867.

[44]M. Malter, "Natural killer cells, vitamins, and other blood components of vegetarian and omnivorous Men," *Nutrition and Cancer*, 12 (1989), pp. 271–278.

[45]J. Nordenstrom, "Decreased chemotaxic and random migration of leukocytes during intralipid infusion," *American Journal of Clinical Nutrition*, 32 (1979), pp. 2416–2422.

[46]R. R. Watson et al, "Effect of beta-carotene on lymphocyte subpopulations in elderly humans," *American Journal of Clinical Nutrition*, 53 (1991), pp. 90–94.

[47]S. Boyd Eaton, M.D., Marjorie Shostak and Melvin Konner, M.D., Ph.D., *The Paleolithic Prescription*, New York: Harper and Row, (1988), p. 86.

[48]L. A. Cohen and E. L. Wynder, "Do dietary monounsaturated fatty acids play a protective role in carcinogenesis and cardiovascular disease?" *Medical Hypotheses*, 31:2 (February 1990), pp. 83–89.

[49]J. J. Vitale and S. A. Broitman, "Lipids and immune function," *Cancer Research*, 41 (September 1981), pp. 3706–3710.

[50]Will Durant, *Our Oriental Heritage*, (1954); *The Life of Greece*, (1939); and *Caesar and Christ*, (1957). New York: Simon and Schuster.

[51]H. D. F. Kitto, *The Greeks*, New York: Penguin Books, (1957), p. 33.

[52]A. Nomura, B. Henderson and J. Lee, "Breast cancer and diet among the Japanese in Hawaii," *American Journal of Clinical Nutrition*, 31:11 (November 1978), pp. 2020–2025.

[53]G. Colditz et al, "Family history, age, and risk of breast cancer. Prospective data from the Nurses' Health Study," *Journal of the American Medical Association*, 270:3 (July 21, 1993), pp. 338–343.

[54]L. Aschoff, "Atherosclerosis," in *Lectures in Pathology*, New York, Hoeber, (1924), p. 131.

[55]H. Beitske, "Zur entsthehung der alherosklerose," *Virchow's Archiv a Pathological Anatomy and Histology*, 267 (1928), pp. 625–647.

[56]M. Hindhede, "The effect of food restriction during war on mortality in Copenhagen," *Journal of the American Medical Association* (February 7, 1920), p. 381.

[57]A. Strom and R. A. Jensen, "Mortality from circulatory diseases in Norway, 1940–1945," *Lancet*, 1 (1951), pp. 126–129.

[58]G. Schettler, "Cardiovascular diseases during and after World War II," *Preventive Medicine*, 8 (1979), pp. 581–590.

[59]F. Berrino and G. Gatta, "Energy-rich diet and breast cancer risk," *International Journal of Cancer*, 44:1 (July 15, 1989), pp. 186–187.

[60]L. J. Vatten and S. Kvinnsland, "Body height and risk of breast cancer: A prospective study of 23,831 Norwegian women," *British Journal of Cancer*, 61 (1990), pp. 881–885.

[61]F. De Waard and D. Trichopoulos, "A unifying concept of the aetiology of breast cancer," *International Journal of Cancer*, 41 (1988), pp. 666–669.

[62]*The Surgeon General's Report on Nutrition and Health*, U.S. Department of Health and Human Services, Publication No. 88-50210, Washington DC, 1988.

## CHAPTER 6 THE ESTROGEN CONNECTION

[63]David Ingram et al, "Obesity and breast disease: the role of female sex hormones," *Cancer*, 64:5 (September 1, 1989), pp. 1049–1053.

[64]D. Heber et al, "Reduction of serum estradiol in postmenopausal women given free access to low-fat high-carbohydrate diet," *Nutrition*, 7:2 (March/April 1991), pp. 137–139.

[65]B. R. Goldin et al, "Estrogen excretion patterns and plasma levels in vegetarian and omnivorous women," *New England Journal of Medicine*, 307:25 (December 16, 1982), pp. 1542–1547.

[66]E. L. Wynder, M.D., "Dietary factors related to breast cancer," *Cancer*, 46, Supplement (August 1980), pp. 899–904.

[67]P. Hill et al, "Prolactin levels in populations at risk for breast cancer," *Cancer Research*, 36:4 (1976), pp. 102–106.

[68]E. L. Wynder, M.D., "The dietary environment and cancer," *Journal of the American Dietetic Association*, 71 (1977), pp. 385–392.

[69]R. E. Hughes, "Hypothesis: a new look at dietary fiber," *Human Nutrition: Clinical Nutrition*, 40:C (1986), pp. 81–86.

[70]D. P. Rose et al, "High-fiber diet reduces serum estrogen concentrations in premenopausal women," *American Journal of Clinical Nutrition*, 54:3 (September 1991), pp. 520–525.

[71]M. C. Pike et al, "Hormones and breast cancer," *Banbury Report*, 8, New York, Cold Springs Harbour Laboratory, (1981), pp. 3–18.

[72]Examiner News Services, "Beefing Up Japan," *San Francisco Examiner*, (June 16, 1993).

[73]Marcia Herman-Giddens, "Girls reaching puberty earlier," *Your Health*, (July 27, 1993), p. 43.

[74]S. Boyd Eaton, Marjorie Shostak and Melvin Konner M.D., PhD., *The Paleolithic Prescription*, New York: Harper and Row, (1988), p. 220.

[75]P. L. Krohn, "Rapid growth, short life," *Journal of the American Medical Association*, 171 (1959), p. 461.

[76]A. N. Exton-Smith, "Physiological aspects of aging: relationship to nutrition," *American Journal of Clinical Nutrition*, 25 (1972), pp. 853–859.

[77]G. T. Beatson, "On the treatment of inoperable cases of carcinoma of the mamma: suggestions for a new method of treatment with illustrative cases," *Lancet*, 2:104–107, (1896), pp. 162–167.

[78]N. A. Lathrop and J. B. Loeb, cited by R. W. Raven in *Cancer*, London, Butterworth & Co. Ltd., (1957), v. 1, p. 5.

[79]Graham Colditz, "Foreward," *Estrogen and Breast Cancer* by Carol Ann Rinzler, New York: Macmillan Publishing Co., (1993), pp. xi–xiv.

[80]K. S. Steinberg et al, "A meta-analysis of the effect of estrogen replacement therapy on the risk of breast cancer", *Journal of the American Medical Association*, 265:15 (April 17, 1991), pp. 1985–1990.

[81]M. D. Bergkvist et al, "The risk of breast cancer after estrogen and estrogen-progestin replacement." *New England Journal of Medicine*, 321:5 (August 3, 1989), pp. 293–297.

[82]J. C. Gallagher et al, "Effect of progestin therapy on cortical and trabecular bone: comparison with estrogen," *American Journal of Medicine*, 90 (1991), pp. 171–178.

[83]A. A. Nabulsi, "Association of hormone-replacement therapy with various cardiovascular risk factors in postmenopausal women," *New England Journal of Medicine*, 328:15 (April 15, 1993), pp. 1069–1075.

[84]P. W. F. Wilson, R. J. Garrison and W. P. Castelli, "Postmenopausal estrogen use, cigarette smoking, and cardiovascular morbidity in women over 50: the Framingham study," *New England Journal of Medicine*, 313 (October 24, 1985), pp. 1038–1043.

[85]M. J. Stampfer et al, "A prospective study of postmenopausal estrogen therapy and coronary heart disease," *New England Journal of Medicine*, 313 (October 24, 1985), pp. 1044–1049.

[86]M. Lock, "Contested meanings of the menopause," *Lancet*, 337 (1991), pp. 1270–1272.

[87]H. Adlercreutz et al, "Dietary phyto-oestrogens and the menopause in Japan," *Lancet*, 339 (May 16, 1992), p. 1233.

## CHAPTER 7    FACTS ABOUT FATS

[88]J. H. Weisburger, "Nutritional approach to cancer prevention with emphasis on vitamins, antioxidants, and carotenoids," *American Journal of Clinical Nutrition*, 53, Supplement (1991), pp. 226s–237s.

[89]D. P. Rose, "Dietary fiber, phytoestrogens, and breast cancer," *Nutrition*, 8:1 (January/February 1992), pp. 47–51.

[90]*Encyclopedia Britannica*, 13, (1974), p. 524.

[91]*Oxford English Dictionary*, 6, (1989), p. 236.

[92]K. Sugiura, *The Publications of Kanematsu Sugiura: Memorial Edition*, 4 volumes, foreword by Chester Stock, New York, Sloan-Kettering Institute, (1965).

[93]K. K. Carroll, "Dietary fats and cancer," *American Journal of Clinical Nutrition*, 53, Supplement (1991), pp. 1064s–1067s.

[94]R. N. Robertson, *The Lively Membranes*, Cambridge, MA: Cambridge University Press, (1983).

[95]J. Barone, "Dietary fat and natural-killer-cell activity," *American Journal of Clinical Nutrition*, 50 (1989), pp. 861–867.

[96]B. Halliwell, "Free radicals: aging and disease," *Annals of Internal Medicine*, 107 (1987), p. 528.

[97]A. T. Diplock, "Antioxidant nutrients and disease prevention: an overview," *American Journal of Clinical Nutrition*, 53, Supplement (1991), pp. 189s–193s.

[98]C. Csillag, and P. Aldhous, "Smoking and Health. Signs of damage by radicals," *Science*, 258 (December 18, 1992), p. 1875.

[99]P. Cerutti, "Proxidant states and tumor production," *Science*, 227 (1985), pp. 375–381.

[100]J. M. Gaziano et al, "Dietary antioxidants and cardiovascular disease," *Annals of the New York Academy of Science*, 669 (1992), pp. 249–259.

[101]G. R. Howe et al, "Dietary factors and risk of breast cancer: combined analysis of 12 case-control studies," *Journal of the National Cancer Institute*, 82 (1990), pp. 561–569.

[102]D. J. Hunter et al, "A prospective study of the intake of vitamins C, E, and A and the risk of breast cancer," *New England Journal of Medicine*, 329:4 (July 22, 1993), pp. 234–240.

[103]S. G. Jenkinson, "Oxygen toxicity," *Intensive Care Medicine*, 3 (1988), pp. 137–152.

[104]M. J. Stampfer et al, "Vitamin E consumption and the risk of coronary disease in women," *New England Journal of Medicine*, 328:20 (May 20, 1993), pp. 1444–1449.

[105]W. C. Willett, "Intake of *trans*-fatty acids and risk of coronary heart disease among women," *Lancet*, 341: 8845 (March 6, 1993), pp. 581–585.

[106]U. Erasmus, *Fats and Oils*, Burnaby, BC, Canada: Alive Books, (1986), Chapter 16, *Trans*-Fatty Acids, p. 100.

[107]L. Kaizer, N. F. Boyd et al, "Fish consumption and breast cancer risk: an ecological study," *Nutrition and Cancer*, 12: 1 (1989), pp. 61–68.

[108]E. L. Wynder, M.D., "Strategies toward the primary prevention of cancer," *Archives of Surgery*, 125 (February, 1990), pp. 163–169.

[109]Jeremy Rifkin, *Beyond Beef*, New York: Dutton, (1992), p. 163.

[110]Michael Klaper, *Vegan Nutrition: Just What the Doctor Ordered*, AHIMSA Videotape No. 12, American Vegan Society, Malaga, New Jersey, (1993).

[111]M. Hindhede, "The effect of food restriction during war on mortality in Copenhagen," *Journal of the American Medical Association*, 74 (6): 381-2 (February 7, 1920).

[112]E. White et al, "Maintenance of a low-fat diet: follow-up of the Women's Health Trial," *Cancer Epidemiology, Biomarkers and Prevention*, 1 (4): 315–22, (1992), (May-June).

[113]F. De Waard, "Breast cancer incidence and nutritional status with particular reference to body weight and height," *Cancer Research*, 35 (1975), p. 3351.

[114]M. B. Wheeler and D. R. Campion, "Animal production—a longstanding biotechnological success," *American Journal of Clinical Nutrition*, 58, Supplement (1993), pp. 276s–281s.

[115]F. Falck, Jr., A. Ricci, M. S. Wolff et al, "Pesticides and polychlorinated biphenyl residues in human breast lipids and their relation to breast cancer," *Archives of Environmental Health*, 47 (March/April 1992), pp. 143–146.

[116]M. Unger et al, "Organochlorine compounds in human breast fat from deceased with and without breast cancer and in a biopsy material from newly diagnosed patients undergoing breast surgery," *Environmental Research*, 34: (1984), pp. 24-28.

[117]M. S. Wolff et al, "Blood levels of organochlorine residues and risk of breast cancer," *Journal of the National Cancer Institute*, 85:8 (April 21, 1993), pp. 648–652.

[118]J. L. Young, "California Cancer Registry, January 1993, Death Records," presented at *Controversies in Breast Cancer* conference, (September 10, 1993), San Francisco.

[119]S. A. Pakeman, *Ceylon*, New York: Frederick A Praeger, (1964), p. 147.

[120]G. L. Cockerell et al, "Seroprevalence of bovine immunodeficiency-like virus and bovine leukemia virus in a dairy cattle herd," *Veterinary Microbiology*, 31:2–3 (June 1, 1992), pp. 109–116.

[121]F. Paradisi et al, "Is fast food toxo-food?" *New England Journal of Medicine*, 313:17, (October 24, 1985), p. 1092.

[122]G. L. Cockerell et al, "Seroprevalence of bovine immunodeficiency-like virus and bovine leukemia virus in a dairy cattle herd," *Veterinary Microbiology*, 31: 2-3 (June 1, 1992), pp. 109–116.

[123]Jacobs R. M. et al, "Detection of multiple retroviral infections in cattle and cross-reactivity of bovine immunodeficiency-like virus," *Canadian Journal of Veterinary Research*, 56(4) (October 1992), pp. 353–359.

[124]T. F. Malivanova and S. V. Litvinov, "Antibodies to retroviruses of types C and D in female patients with benign and malignant mammary tumors," *Acta Virologica*, 34(1):19–26 (February 1990), p. 26.

[125]J. W. Wilesmith, J. B. Ryan and W. D. Hueston, "Case control studies of calf feeding practices and meat and bonemeal inclusion in proprietary concentrates," *Research in Veterinary Science*, 52:3 (May 1992), pp. 325–331.

[126]A. S. Cunningham, "Lymphomas and Animal-Protein Consumption," *Lancet*, 2: 7996 (November 27, 1976), p. 1184.

[127]G. Ursin, et al, "Milk consumption and cancer incidence: a Norwegian prospective study," *British Journal of Cancer*, 61:3 (March 1990), pp. 456–459.

[128]D. W. Cramer, "Lactose persistence and milk consumption as determinants of ovarian cancer risk," *American Journal of Epidemiology*, 130:5 (November 1989), pp. 904–910.

[129]P. Mills et al, "Dietary habits and breast cancer incidence among Seventh-Day Adventists," *Cancer*, 79, (1989), pp. 465–471.

[130]T. Hirayama, "Epidemiology of breast cancer with special reference to the role of diet," *Journal of Preventive Medicine*, 7:173–174 (1978).

## CHAPTER 8   THE EXERCISE FACTOR

[131]R. S. Paffenbarger, W. E. Hale, "Work activity and coronary heart mortality," *New England Journal of Medicine*, 292 (1975), pp. 545–550.

[132]R. S. Paffenbarger et al, "The influence of physical activity on the incidence of site-specific cancers in college alumni," *Advances in Experimental Medicine and Biology*, 322 (1992), pp. 7–15.

[133]S. Blair, "Physical fitness and all-cause mortality," *Journal of the American Medical Association*, 262:issue (November 3, 1989), pp. 2395–2401.

[134]A. P. Simopoulus, "Energy imbalance and cancer of the breast, colon and prostate," *Medical Oncology and Tumor Pharmacotherapy*, 7:2–3 (1990), pp 109–120.

[135]N. F. Boyd and V. McGuire, "Evidence of association between plasma high-density lipoprotein cholesterol and risk factors for breast cancer," *Journal of the National Cancer Institute*, 82:6 (March 21, 1990), pp. 460–468.

[136]D. Albanes, A. Blair and P. R. Taylor, "Physical activity and risk of cancer in the NHANES I population," *American Journal of Public Health*, 79:6 (June 1989), pp. 744–750.

[137]R. E. Frisch et al, "Magnetic resonance imaging of body fat of athletes compared with controls, and the oxidative metabolism of estradiol," *Metabolism: Clinical and Experimental*, 41:2 (February 1992), pp. 191–193.

[138]R. E. Frisch, G. Wyshak, N. L. Albright et al, "Lower prevalence of breast cancer and cancers of the reproductive system among former college athletes compared to non-athletes," *British Journal of Cancer*, 52 (1985), pp. 885–891.

[139]R. E. Frisch et al, "Lower prevalence of non-reproductive system cancers among female former college athletes," *Medicine & Science in Sports & Exercise*, 21:3 (1989), pp. 250–253.

[140]L. Bernstein, R. K. Ross and B. E. Henderson, "Prospects for the primary care of breast cancer," *American Journal of Epidemiology*, 135:2 (January 15, 1992), pp. 142–152.

[141]J. Ritz, "The role of natural killer cells in immune surveillance," *New England Journal of Medicine*, 320:26 (1989), pp. 1748–1749.

[142]L. T. Mackinnon, "Exercise and natural killer cells: what is the relationship?" *Sports Medicine*, 7:3 (1989), pp. 141–149.

[143]L. A. Cohen et al, "Modulation of N-nitrosomethylurea induced mammary tumorigenesis by dietary fat and voluntary exercise," *In Vivo*, 5:4 (July/August 1991), pp. 333–344.

[144]M. L. Winningham et al, *Oncology Nursing Forum*, 16:5 (September/October 1989), pp. 683–689.

[145]J. E. Vena et al, "Lifetime occupational exercise and colon cancer," *American Journal of Epidemiology*, 122 (1985), pp. 357–365.

## CHAPTER 9   IT'S NEVER TOO LATE TO START

[146]E. L. Wynder et al, "A comparison of survival rates between American and Japanese patients with breast cancer," *Surgery, Gynecology and Obstetrics*, 117 (1963), pp. 196–200.

[147]L. E. Holm et al, "Treatment failure and dietary habits in women with breast cancer," *Journal of the National Cancer Institute*, 85:1 (January 6, 1993), pp. 32–36.

[148]N. F. Boyd, "Nutrition and breast cancer," *Journal of the National Cancer Institute*, 85:1 (January 6, 1993), pp. 6–7.

[149]David Gregorio et al, "Dietary fat consumption and survival among women with breast cancer," *Journal of the National Cancer Institute*, 75:1 (July 1985), pp. 37–41.

[150]John A. McDougall, "Preliminary study of diet as an adjunct therapy for breast cancer" *Journal Breast*, 10:1 (1984), pp. 18–21.

[151]Ruth Heidrich, Ph.D., *A Race for Life; From Cancer to the Ironman*, 1415 Victoria St., Honolulu, Hawaii, (1990).

[152]René Verreault, "Dietary fat in relation to prognostic Indicators in breast cancer," *Journal of the National Cancer Institute*, 80:11 (August 3, 1988), pp. 818–825.

[153]S. C. Newman et al, "A study of the effect of weight and dietary fat on breast cancer survival time," *American Journal of Epidemiology*, 123:5 (May 1986), pp. 764–767.

[154]A. P. Boyar et al, "Response to a diet low in total fat in women with postmenopausal breast cancer: a pilot study," *Nutrition and Cancer*, 11:2 (1988), pp. 93–99

[155]A. Morabia and E. L. Wynder, "Epidemiology and natural history of breast cancer. Implications for the body weight–breast cancer controversy," *Surgical Clinics of North America*, 70:4, (August 1990), pp. 739–752.

[156]Gary Meadows, "Diet changes may buy cancer patients time," *Science News*, 142 (November 21, 1992), p. 324.

## CHAPTER 10    THE BREAST-CANCER-PREVENTION FOOD PLAN

[157]G. Block et al, "Fruit, vegetables and cancer prevention: a review of the epidemiologic evidence," *Nutrition and Cancer*, 18 (1992), pp. 1–29.

[158]Carl Lewis, Radio Interview, KST, 650 AM Radio, Sacramento, May 12, 1993.

[159]B. J. Abelow et al, "Cross-cultural association between dietary animal protein and hip fracture: a hypothesis," *Calcified Tissue International*, 50:1 (January 1992), pp. 14–18.

[160]B. Armstrong and R. Doll, "Environmental factors and cancer incidence and mortality in different countries with special reference to dietary practices," *International Journal of Cancer*, 15 (1975), pp. 617–631.

[161]G. Hems, "The contributions of diet and childbearing to breast-cancer rates," *British Journal of Cancer*, 37, pp. 947–982.

## CHAPTER 11    GETTING STARTED: SAMPLE MEAL PLANS

[162]T. Chou, "Wake up and smell the coffee," *Western Journal of Medicine*, 157 (November 1992), pp. 544–553.

[163]J. Pawlega, "Breast cancer and smoking, vodka drinking and dietary habits. A case-control study," *Acta Oncologica*, 31: 4 (1992), pp. 387–392.

[164]M. Ewertz, "Alcohol consumption and breast cancer risk in Denmark," *Cancer Causes and Control*, 2:4 (July 1991), pp. 247–252.

[165]G. G. Meadows et al, "Ethanol induces marked suppression of lymphocyte populations as well as natural killer cell activity in mice," *Alcoholism*, 16:3 (June 1992), pp. 474–479.

[166]M. E. Reichman et al, "Effects of alcohol consumption on plasma and urinary hormone concentrations in premenopausal women," *Journal of the National Cancer Institute*, 85:9 (May 5, 1993), pp. 692–727.

[167]John A. McDougall, M.D., *The McDougall Program: Twelve Days to Dynamic Health*, New York: NAL Books, (1990), p. 44.

[168]R. D. Mattes, "Fat preference and adherence to a reduced-fat diet," *American Journal of Clinical Nutrition*, 57 (1993), pp. 373–381.

## CHAPTER 13    THE KRADJIAN GUIDE TO RESTAURANT EATING

[169]Anon, "Whose meal is it, anyway?" *Tufts University Diet and Nutrition Letter*, 11:3 (May 1993), p. 1.

## CHAPTER 15    FOR DOCTORS ONLY

[170]P. G. Toniolo, "Calorie-providing nutrients and risk of breast cancer," *Journal of the National Cancer Institute*, 81:4 (February 15, 1989), pp. 278–286.

[171]L. A. Cohen, D. P. Rose and E. L. Wynder, "A rationale for dietary intervention in postmenopausal breast cancer," *Nutrition and Cancer* 19:1 (1993), pp. 1–10.

## Appendix I    Harvard and the Harvard Nurses' Study

[172]Michael Lagios, M.D., Department of Pathology, California Pacific Medical Center, San Francisco, California. Personal communication. September 21, 1993.

[173]S. Kikuchi et al, "A case control study of breast cancer, mammary cyst and dietary, drinking or smoking habit in Japan," *Japanese Journal of Cancer Clinics*, Special Issue (February 1990), pp. 365–369.

[174]A. Morabia, "Reproducibility of food frequency measurements and inferences from a case control study," *Epidemiology*, 1:4 (July 1990), pp. 305–310.

[175]A. P. Boyar et al, "Recommendations for the prevention of chronic disease: the application for breast disease," *American Journal of Clinical Nutrition*, 48:3 Supplement (September 1988), pp. 896–900.

[176]A. P. Boyar et al, "Response to a diet low in total fat in women with postmenopausal breast cancer: a pilot study," *Nutrition and Cancer* 11:2 (1988), pp. 93–99.

[177]A. R. Kristal et al, "Long-term maintenance of a low-fat diet: durability of fat-related habits in the Woman's Health Trial," *Journal of the American Dietetic Association*, 92:5 (May 1992), pp. 553–559.

[178]B. Kronman, *San Francisco Chronicle*, (October 21, 1992).

[179]W. C. Willett et al, "Dietary fat and the risk of breast cancer," *New England Journal of Medicine*, 316 (January 1, 1987), pp. 22–28.

[180]Ross Prentice, "Letters to the Editor," *Journal of the American Medical Association*, 269:14 (April 14, 1993), pp. 1790–1791.

[181]E. L. Wynder, L. Cohen and S. Stellman, "Letters to the Editor," *Journal of the American Medical Association*, 269:14 (April 14, 1993), pp. 1791.

[182]*Physician's Weekly*, 10:15 (April 26, 1993).

[183]A. Morabia and E. L. Wynder, "Epidemiology and natural history of breast cancer, implications for the body weight-breast cancer controversy," *Surgical Clinics of North America*, 70:4 (August 1990), pp. 739–752.

[184]P. J. Goodwin and N. F. Boyd, "Body size and breast cancer prognosis: a critical review of the evidence," *Breast Cancer Research and Treatment*, 3 (October 16, 1990), pp. 205–214.

[185]G. R. Howe et al, "Dietary factors and risk of breast cancer: Combined analysis of 12 case-control studies," *Journal of the National Cancer Institute*, 82 (1990), pp. 561–569.

[186]G. R. Howe, "High-fat diets and breast cancer risk: the epidemiologic evidence," *Journal of the American Medical Association*, 268:15 (October 21, 1992), pp. 2080–2081.

## APPENDIX 2    RESEARCH FUNDING: AN INCENTIVE FOR BIAS

[187]D. Blumenthal, "Academic-industry relationships in the life sciences," *Journal of the American Medical Association*, Vol. 268:23 (December 16, 1992), pp. 3344–3349.

[188]D. Blumenthal et al, "University-industry research relationships in biotechnology: implications for the university," *Science*, 232:4756 (June 13, 1986), pp. 1361–1366.

[189]J. D. Dingell, "Shattuck Lecture," *New England Journal of Medicine*, 328:22 (June 3, 1993), pp. 1610–1636.

[190]K. J. Rothman, "Conflict of interest, the new McCarthyism in science," *Journal of the American Medical Association*, 269: 21 (June 2, 1993), pp. 2782–2784.

[191]J. P. Kassirer, "Medicine at center stage," *New England Journal of Medicine*, 328:17 (April 29, 1993), pp. 1268–90.

[192]A. S. Relman, *New England Journal of Medicine*, 320:14 (April 6, 1989), pp. 933–934.

[193]Fredrick J. Stare, M.D., *Adventures in Nutrition*, Hanover, MA: Christopher Publishing House, (1991).

[194]David Steinman, *Diet for a Poisoned Planet*, New York: Harmony Books, (1990).

[195]F. J. Stare, R. E. Olson, and E. M. Whelan, *Balanced Nutrition Beyond the Cholesterol Scare*, Bob Adams, Inc., Holbrook, MA, (1989), pp. 360.

# Resource Guide

The following books will help you implement the dietary plan described in this book. Some recipes may require modification to meet our guidelines. Books are listed alphabetically by author.

Barnard, Neal D., M.D., *Food for Life: How the New Four Food Groups Can Save Your Life*. New York: Harmony Books, 1993. Nicely written and presented explanation of the latest nutritional information. Recipes and menus provided.

Bortz, Walter M. II, M.D., *We Live Too Short and Die Too Long*. New York: Bantam Books, 1991. An inspirational guide to living longer and better. Strong emphasis on the importance of exercise.

Carper, Jean, *Food—Your Miracle Medicine*. New York: HarperCollins Publishers, 1993. A helpful review of food as it relates to health.

Connor, Sonja L., M.S., R.D. and William E., M.D., *The New American Diet*. New York: Simon and Schuster, 1986. Very nice people, and a very nice book. The 20-percent-fat diet described is a bit higher in fat than I recommend, but adaptations can be easily made. Recipes included.

Love, Susan M., M.D., *Dr. Susan Love's Breast Book*. Massachusetts: Addison-Wesley Publishing Company, Inc. 1990. Excellent general information on the subject of breast cancer diagnosis and treatment. Not intended as a primer on prevention.

McDougall, John A., M.D., and Mary, *The McDougall Program: Twelve Days to Dynamic Health*. New York: Plume, 1990. A description of the twelve-day, live-in program that the McDougalls have used to help thousands. Recipes included.

McDougall, John A., M.D., and Mary, *The New McDougall Cookbook*. New York: E. P. Dutton, 1993. Eight-to-10-percent fat, nondairy, nonoil, vegetarian recipes. You'll be amazed at how good many are.

McDougall, John A., M.D., *The McDougall Program for Maximum Weight Loss*. New York: E. P. Dutton, 1994. Additional recipes for low-fat eating.

Moran, Victoria, *Get the Fat Out: 501 Simple Ways to Cut the Fat in Any Diet*. New York: Crown Trade Paperbacks, 1994. Dozens of practical tips and a great deal of good information on how to implement a health-promoting, anticancer diet. Recipes included.

Ornish, Dean, M.D., *Dr. Dean Ornish's Program for Reversing Heart Disease*. New York: Random House, 1990. Similar to the above, but oriented more toward cardiac disease than to weight loss. Excellent general explanation of modern life-extension nutrition. Recipes included.

Ornish, Dean, M.D., *Eat More, Weigh Less*. New York: HarperCollins Publishers, 1993. Although a weight-loss book, the dietary advice is very close to mine and nicely presented by a pioneer in scientific nutrition. Nonfat milk products are allowed in the recipes for this plan.

Pritikin, Robert, *The New Pritikin Program*. New York: Simon and Schuster, 1990. The latest in the pioneering series started by the late Nathan Pritikin. Good, practical exposition and meal plans with recipes. Includes nonfat milk products and lean meats. Includes recipes.

Wagner, Lindsay and Ariane Spade, *The High Road to Health: A Vegetarian Cookbook*. New York: Prentice-Hall Press, 1990. Helpful tips and creative recipes. They do use a bit of oil.

# Index

## ROBERT M. KRADJIAN, M.D.—BREAST SURGEON

After 30 years in the practice of surgery, Dr. Kradjian has concluded that nutrition is the key to the breast cancer problem in America. His extensive study of the world's scientific and medical literature has reinforced his belief that most breast cancers can be prevented. Currently Chief of General Surgery at Seton Medical Center in Daly City, California, Dr. Kradjian holds a B.A. in Psychology from the University of California at Los Angeles and earned his medical degree from the University of California at San Francisco. He is certified by the American Board of Surgery and has served as Chief of Surgery on the hospital ship S.S. *Hope* in Colombia, Sri Lanka, and Tunisia. As a volunteer surgeon he has worked in Vietnam, India, and Thailand.

Dr. Kradjian coauthored the medical text *Renal Carcinoma* by W. B. Saunders in 1967 and has authored fifteen patient education booklets. He has been featured on radio and television programs regarding breast cancer prevention, detection, and treatment, and he lectures on a regular basis. Dr. Kradjian and his wife, Christine, have been married for 26 years and live in the San Francisco Bay Area.

# SAVE YOURSELF FROM BREAST CANCER

1. EIGHTY PERCENT OF AMERICAN WOMEN WITH BREAST CANCER HAVE NO BLOOD RELATIVES WITH THAT DISEASE.

2. BREAST CANCER IS RARE IN COUNTRIES WHERE WOMEN EAT LOW-FAT DIETS. THESE WOMEN ARE "PROTECTED." IN AMERICA, BREAST CANCER IS COMMON AND INCREASING. WOMEN EAT HIGH-FAT DIETS AND ARE NOT PROTECTED.

3. WHEN WOMEN FROM THE "PROTECTED" COUNTRIES MOVE TO THE "UNPROTECTED" COUNTRIES, THEY LOSE THEIR PROTECTION. THEREFORE, THAT PROTECTION IS NOT GENETIC, IT IS ENVIRONMENTAL.

4. EARLY DETECTION, TREATMENT, AND RESEARCH HAVE NOT SOLVED THE BREAST CANCER PROBLEM IN AMERICA.

5. PREVENTION OF BREAST CANCER IS INFINITELY BETTER THAN EARLY DETECTION. TOO OFTEN, BREAST CANCER CAN SPREAD BEFORE IT CAN BE DETECTED.

6. A LOW-FAT, HIGH-FIBER, PLANT-BASED DIET GREATLY REDUCES THE RISK OF BREAST CANCER. *EAT* WHOLE GRAINS, POTATOES, RICE, CORN, BEANS, VEGETABLES, AND FRUIT. *AVOID* MEAT, SATURATED FATS, MOST OILS, MILK, EGGS, CHEESE, AND ALCOHOL.

**EMPOWER YOURSELVES.
TAKE CHARGE OF YOUR HEALTH AND
YOUR FUTURE.**